EVERYTHING YOU NEED TO KNOW
ABOUT CONTACT LENSES

Dr R.M. YOUNGSON is a Consultant Ophthalmic Surgeon, with many years' experience in fitting contact lenses to all kinds of patients. He is a member of the Faculty of Ophthalmology at the Royal College of Surgeons, and has published numerous articles on the subject of ophthalmology. He is currently writing a popular guide to eyes and common eye diseases. He is married, with five children.

D1098547

Overcoming Common Problems Series

Overcoming Common Problems Series

Overcoming Common Problems

EVERYTHING YOU NEED TO KNOW ABOUT CONTACT LENSES

Dr R.M. Youngson

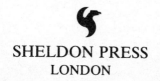

SHELDON PRESS
LONDON

First published in Great Britain in 1984 by
Sheldon Press, SPCK, Marylebone Road, London NW1 4DU

Copyright © R.M. Youngson 1984

British Library Cataloguing in Publication Data
Youngson, R.M.
  Everything you need to know about contact
  lenses.—(Overcoming common problems)
  1. Contact lenses
  I. Title   II. Series
  617.7'523   RE997.C6

ISBN 0–85969–458–5
ISBN 0–85969–459–3 Pbk

Typeset by Inforum Ltd, Portsmouth
Printed in Great Britain by
Richard Clay (The Chaucer Press) Ltd,
Bungay, Suffolk

Contents

Preface

Millions of people are now enjoying all the advantages of contact lenses – better vision, greater convenience and improved appearance – but there are still many spectacle wearers who, having considered contact lenses, are deterred from trying them by all sorts of fears and fancies. Most of these are the result of lack of knowledge of what contact lenses are all about. There are also many who have obtained contact lenses but, for a variety of reasons, have experienced problems. To both of these groups, this little book is dedicated.

R.M. Youngson, 1984

1

A Look Around The Eye

To understand contact lenses properly it is helpful to have some idea of how the eye works. This brief chapter will tell you all you need to know.

The eye is rather like a TV camera – its job is to focus a sharp image, of whatever it is pointed at, on to a special screen, the retina. This, in turn, converts the image into a sequence of electrical signals which are carried out of the back of each eye by a cable called the optic nerve.

The process of seeing

The actual experience of seeing is not understood, but we do know that the optic nerves are connected to a part of the brain at the back of the head and that if this part of the brain is destroyed vision will be lost, even if the eyes are completely normal. The way in which the conscious image is formed – what we are experiencing when we say that we are 'seeing' must be somewhat similar to what happens in a TV receiver when the electrical signal from the aerial is transformed into a picture. But this activity is quite remote from the function of the eyes themselves.

Although the eye is just the first stage in the process of seeing, it is, however, the stage which most commonly goes wrong so, again, it is useful to know a little about it.

The eye-ball is an approximately spherical globe, about one inch in diameter, with a rather prominent bulge (called the cornea) on the front made of a perfectly transparent material. This lens is kept constantly wetted by a salt solution produced by hundreds of tiny glands in the membrane (the conjunctiva) which lines the lids, covers the white of the eye and seals the spaces between the insides of the lids and the eyeball. Because they are thus sealed the fear of many people contemplating contact lenses – that a lens may slip round behind the eye – is groundless.

Whenever the cornea begins to dry, an automatic blinking action causes the insides of the eye-lids to sweep across the surface of the cornea, renewing the tear film and restoring its efficiency.

The most important part of the cornea, in connection with contact lenses, is the outer skin (the epithelium). It is especially sensitive to lack of oxygen (which it gets directly from the air, through the tear film) and if deprived for more than about four hours, will die and strip off, leaving the very sensitive deeper layer of the cornea exposed – an extremely painful condition. Fortunately, the epithelium has an extraordinary ability to grow again very rapidly. Under ideal conditions it grows in about a day – but that will be a very painful day for the person concerned and he or she will hardly be able to open the damaged eye. However, if you treat the epithelium with due respect and use your contact lenses correctly, you should never have this problem.

Behind the cornea is a shallow chamber full of water, bounded behind by the iris – which gives the eye its colour. At the centre of the iris is a circular hole, the pupil, which changes size according to the brightness of the light entering the eye – rather like a shutter. Very bright light causes the pupil to become quite small and in the dark it becomes very large. Immediately behind the iris is the internal 'crystalline' lens responsible for fine focusing so that one can look from distant objects to near ones and still get a clear image.

The retina (which lines the whole of the inside of the back of the eye), is composed of light-sensitive cells and inter-connecting nerve – fibres which perform the important function of impro-ving the contrast and sharpness of edges. The output connections from the retina join at the back of the eye to form the optic nerve connecting the eye to the brain.

In the upper and outer part of each eye socket is the lacrimal gland, which produces tears during emotion or when the eye is irritated by a foreign body such as a contact lens or by smoke, wind etc. Normally, the cornea and conjunctiva are kept moist by tears from the small conjunctive glands already mentioned, but if additional wetting is required, the lacrimal glands come into action. Excess tears tend to overflow and run down the face, but near the inner end of each lid there is a little opening from which a tube runs down into the back of the nose. This tube carries away excess tears so you may well find you need to blow your nose more than usual when first you try contact lenses. Your fitter will have a supply of tissues ready.

Now let us consider why people need contact lenses.

2

Light, Lenses, Images and Eggs

So let's take a look at this business of lenses. The word comes from the latin word for a lentil and most lenses do look very like a transparent half pea.

We can learn quite a lot about how they work by using a lens to focus the light rays from the sun on to a piece of paper. Because of the distance of the sun, the light rays reaching the lens are, for practical purposes, parallel to each other – this applies to rays from any point more than about six metres or so away. As soon as the rays reach the lens they are bent inwards, forming a small blurred circle on the paper and if you move the paper back and forward, you will find a position in which the circle is sharp and its size least. For any particular lens, the distance from lens to paper, when the image is sharp, is called the 'focal length' of the lens. This little test demonstrates that if the focal length of a person's cornea is not exactly right for the distance from the cornea to the retina, that person will have blurred vision.

Short sight and long sight

The commonest reason for wearing contact lenses is short sight (myopia) and this is the condition in which the focal length of the cornea is too short for the length of the eye. Also, the curve of the cornea is a little too steep, so the corneal lens is too strong and produces a blurred image of distant objects. However, a short-sighted person can see perfectly clearly if the object he is looking at is near the eye; that is why the condition is called 'short sight'.

The degree of myopia (short sight) varies considerably from

4

person to person. Someone who is only very slightly short-sighted may see everything clearly out to a distance of about 4 metres or so, but a very short-sighted person will have to bring the print (or whatever he is trying to see) very close to his eyes – possibly to just a few centimetres.

People who are not short-sighted (these are people whose corneas have the correct focal length) will have crystal clear vision for distant objects. But what happens when they look at near things? Well, if nothing else changes, the vision will be quite blurred. Fortunately, we are provided with an extra lens, inside each eye, programmed to alter its shape automatically in order to fine-focus when necessary.

In older people, these fine-focusing internal lenses become rigid and gradually lose their youthful ability to change shape. Although the distance vision will be perfectly clear and sharp, all near objects – especially print – will be extremely blurred and they will need reading glasses for clear near vision.

The internal focusing lens is of no help to short-sighted people – in fact, focusing with this lens will only make matters worse for them.

Long-sighted people have corneas that are not curved strongly enough. Unlike the myopes however, they can do something about it. If they focus the eyes as if they were looking at something close the vision will at once become clear. So long as the degree of long-sight is not excessive and they are fairly young, they can do this unconsciously. There are millions of young people around who are quite unaware of the fact that they are long-sighted. Sooner or later, however, as the internal lenses gradually harden with age, it becomes more difficult for them to get near objects into focus, and the nearest point of clear vision gradually becomes further and further away until glasses become necessary, first for close work, then for distance. Patients in this situation often say to me, jokingly, that their arms are not long enough.

Long-sight is about as common as short-sight but because long-sight tends to be concealed in this way, the great majority of

5

people wearing contact lenses are short-sighted.

What can be done

As we have seen, the basic problem with short-sighted people is that the cornea acts as a lens which is too strong. If we could arrange for the front surface of the cornea to have a flatter curve, then an exact focus could be achieved.

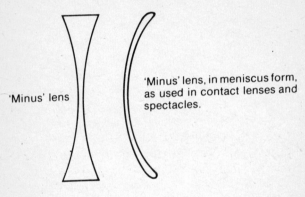

'Minus' lens

'Minus' lens, in meniscus form, as used in contact lenses and spectacles.

Figure 1

There is, fortunately, a simple way of flattening the curve of the front lens of the eye. If we apply to the cornea a tiny, thin plastic lens carefully designed so that the surface in contact with the eye fits the cornea perfectly, and the front surface of this lens has a slightly flatter curve than the cornea has, the image seen by the eye can be made perfectly clear for distance vision and the patient can focus, in the normal way, for near. The contact lens we have designed in this way is actually a bit thinner in the centre than at the edges. When you first see such a lens, you may consider this to be a rather strange shape (see Figure 1) but, as the conventional lens formed by the cornea is too strong, what we need is a negative lens to make it weaker. Lenses of this shape are, in fact, called negative (or 'minus') lenses. All lenses used to

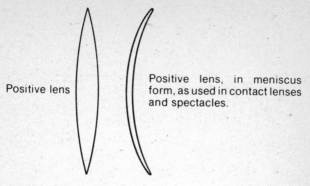

Positive lens

Positive lens, in meniscus form, as used in contact lenses and spectacles.

Figure 2

correct short-sight, whether contact lenses or in spectacles, are of this type – thinner in the centre than at the edge. Lentil-shaped lenses, used in long-sight and as reading glasses, are called positive lenses (see Figure 2).

This way of correcting the focus of short-sighted eyes has a number of major advantages over the more conventional system of putting the negative lenses into a spectacle frame, and the more short-sighted the person concerned, the more marked these advantages become. For a start, an optical system containing several lenses will only work properly if the centres of the various lenses are in a straight line. Since contact lenses move with the eye, they meet this requirement, but this is not so with glasses. Indeed, vision through the edges of strong spectacle lenses produces so much distortion and displacement of the image that the field of clear vision may be severely limited. When a severely short-sighted person is fitted with contact lenses, the improvement in the width of the field of clear vision is so great that such patients nearly always express surprise and delight. 'It's like getting a new pair of eyes!' they will say.

Secondly, the distance of the correcting lens from the eye has an effect on the size of the image; the further away from the eye, the smaller the object being looked at will appear to be. So contact lenses give an obvious advantage in that the reduction in

7

size of the image is less than with glasses.

One of the things spectacle-wearing people often find very annoying is that spectacle lenses require frequent cleaning and polishing. Contact lenses score a point there, as they enjoy the benefit of a built-in windscreen washer and wiper system. Contact lenses, when in use, are automatically kept completely wet at all times (see Chapter 1) and any tendency to surface contamination can be cleared immediately and automatically, simply by blinking.

Astigmatism

The word astigmatism is used to describe a lens that cannot focus a round spot of light to give a small round image. Instead, an astigmatic lens causes an image of the spot which is 'smeared' – blurred and elongated. The lenses I have described so far, whether positive or negative, have a curvature that is the same, whichever diameter we look at. Astigmatic lenses have a different curvature in different diameters. If you find this hard to understand, think of an egg lying on a table and with a circle drawn on its side, as in Figure 3. Obviously, the curve A to B is flatter than the curve C to D; the curve E to F has a steepness somewhere between the two.

The circle on the side of the egg has an astigmatic surface and

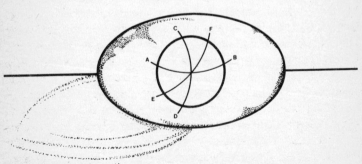

Figure 3 The astigmatic egg.

if a person's cornea is this shape (millions of people's corneas *are* shaped like this) and we want to give him – or her – clear vision, we have a problem. An ordinary positive or negative spherical lens is capable of correcting the error due to one of the curves but can do nothing for the other. What is needed is a lens that has two different degrees of curvature, each correcting the error in its own direction. This is what is done if astigmatism is corrected by spectacle lenses. But, fortunately, most people with astigmatism have it to quite a limited degree and, in these cases, contact lenses can score, in another way, over glasses.

So long as the astigmatism is not severe, a hard contact lens can give perfect vision. However, a soft lens will tend to mould itself to the surface of the cornea, reproducing the irregular shape on its front surface, so that the eye remains astigmatic, although usually to a lesser extent than before.

Accommodation

The last point we have to consider is the way in which we change the focus of the eye in order to see clearly when looking at near objects. To do this we use a faculty we call 'accommodation'. A similar sort of thing occurs when we are using a camera to focus sharply on a near object. We 'accommodate' the lens to the new distance by screwing it outwards so that it is further from the film. The human eye, as I mentioned earlier, has a lens inside it, just behind the pupil, which is actually capable of becoming more sharply curved when necessary. The process is quite automatic and unconscious and works very well in young people but, unfortunately, as we get older the elasticity of our internal lenses becomes less and, around the age of sixty, is lost altogether. This is why older people need glasses for reading, even if the distance vision is perfect. At this stage, a short-sighted person can often get by satisfactorily simply by taking off his glasses. If he wears contact lenses he will need to use reading glasses on top of the contacts, as he is then in the situation of a normal-sighted person. Young people with short sight and wearing contact lenses have no problems – they simply accommodate in the normal way.

Interestingly enough, long-sighted people who are beginning to have close vision problems (this occurs at an earlier age in the long-sighted than in the normal) and who decide to try contact lenses, find that they can manage both distant and near vision much better, and to a more advanced age, than when they use glasses. Short-sighted people wearing contact lenses however, may find that they need reading glasses at a somewhat earlier age than normal.

3

About Short Sight

Because the great majority of contact lens wearers are short-sighted, I thought it would be useful to spend a little more time on this interesting subject, and to deal with some of the many misunderstandings and superstitions connected with it.

Strangely enough, I have found that many short-sighted patients are confused about the correct name for their condition; some even believe that they are 'long-sighted'! So let's start by clarifying what is meant by the term. Short-sighted, or myopic, people are those who cannot see distant objects clearly but can see clearly things that are close. A slightly short-sighted person will see, quite clearly, within two or three metres but may find a distant face a little too blurred to be recognizable. A severely short-sighted person will have to bring an object quite close to his eyes in order to see it clearly.

One thing the short-sighted person can do to improve distant vision is to screw up the muscles round his eyes so that the gap between his lids becomes very narrow. Throughout the ages, short-sighted people have discovered that bunching up the muscles round the eyelids in this way can help and it is from this habit that the name 'myopia' is derived. 'Myopia' means 'muscular' vision. Many myopic people make use of this fact, from time to time, especially in bright conditions, and some have even found that they can get clear distant vision by looking through a small hole in a piece of card. So, if you see somebody with their eyes tightly screwed up and gazing into the distance you will very probably be right if you suspect that they are short-sighted. This can be quite a useful aid to distant vision.

Some common misconceptions

As explained in Chapter 2, short sight is in no sense a disease. It is merely the result of the eyes being slightly longer from front to back, than the focal length of the lens system. In other words, the curvature of the cornea is too great for the length of the eye. When the short-sighted person looks at a distant object the image comes to a focus in front of the retina. When he looks at something near, because light rays entering the eyes are spreading out more, they will focus further back and may reach the retina.

From this, you will see that short-sight could not possibly be caused by reading with the book close to the eyes in childhood, as is commonly believed. As a matter of fact, reading with the book close to your eyes is quite a useful exercise, both of the focusing mechanism of the eyes and of the convergence (ability to turn the eyes inward) and children should not be discouraged from doing this. The reason why close reading was thought to cause short sight was simply that many children, before they were known to be short-sighted, were observed holding their books very close to their faces. They did this, of course, because they were short-sighted.

Another common misconception is that short sight (or just poor vision, generally) can be caused when we try to read in conditions of dim light – as when children read comics under bedclothes with a torch, for instance. There has never been any evidence that the eyes can be injured by doing this; there is even some indication that the visual performance can be improved by regular attempts to discriminate detail in poor light.

The lens and retinal system of the eye cannot be damaged by excessive use, nor can we preserve vision by not using the eyes. Indeed, one form of untreatable visual loss occurs in children who, for one reason or another, fail to use one eye during their early years. This is called 'amblyopia' and nothing can be done to improve it after the age of about eight. Fortunately, however, if such cases are detected early, the vision may be brought to normal.

It is also commonly believed that short sight may be caused by the failure to wear necessary glasses in childhood. I have heard many patients say 'Of course, I ruined my eyes because I wouldn't wear my glasses.' This, too, is a fallacy. Neither the length of the eye nor the curvature of the cornea could be affected in this way. Again, many people think that eyes can be 'ruined' by wearing the wrong glasses. Probably, the origin of this belief is that inaccurate lenses may cause a sense of eye strain by forcing the wearer to focus the eyes unduly. But doing this cannot alter the dimensions of the eyes, or weaken the focusing power.

Heredity factor

The question of heredity in myopia is interesting. There is a fairly strong tendency for short-sighted parents to have short-sighted children. If both father and mother are short-sighted, there is a distinct probability that the children, or some of them, will also be short-sighted. If only one parent is short-sighted there is still a higher than average probability that one or more children will also be affected.

This is not really surprising. If you consider that the basis of family resemblance is in large part, the relative dimensions of the face, the size of the nose, the separation of the eyes, the length of the upper lip and so on) and bearing in mind that short sight is a matter of the dimensions of the eyes, it will appear perfectly logical that children tend to inherit the eye focusing errors of their parents.

Progression of short sight

Short sight commonly begins at about puberty and the degree progresses while body growth is progressing. In ninety-nine cases out of a hundred the progression of the myopia then stops. Many people worry that they will go on becoming more and more short-sighted indefinitely. Fortunately, this is very rare. The degree to which the condition progresses seems to depend largely on the age at which it starts. Thus, the great majority (who don't show any sign of short-sight until the age of twelve or thirteen) are very unlikely to become high myopes. Most will end up with between two and five dioptres of short sight. (The dioptre is the unit of strength of the lens needed to correct the focus of the eye – see Glossary.) But a child who shows significant myopia at the age of, say, three years, will probably progress to a fairly high degree of myopia.

It has often been stated that if contact lenses are fitted during early adolescence, the progress of myopia may be checked. Regrettably, this is not correct. It is perfectly true that growing young myopes require changes of contact lenses much less often than they require changes of glasses – indeed it is quite uncommon for contact lenses to have to be changed at all. But the reason for this is not that the myopia is not progressing, but that any change in the curvature of the cornea becomes irrelevant if hard lenses are being worn (see Chapter 2). In fact, hard lenses tend to 'mould' the corneas so that, while they are being worn, the corneal curvature remains constant. Therefore, the hope of preventing myopia from progressing is *not* a good reason for putting young myopes into contact lenses.

This brings me to the question of the best age at which to start wearing contact lenses. There is no hard and fast answer to this. Much depends on the degree of responsibility of the child and the standard of supervision by the parents. It is as well to bear in mind that, unless carefully watched, most young people will not exercise the degree of care in maintaining the standards of cleanliness and restriction of wearing-time necessary for safety. Except in special cases, such as high myopia or after removal of cataracts present at birth (see Chaper 9), it is probably wise not to begin until about the age of sixteen.

4

What Happens at a Lens Fitting

This chapter describes a typical contact lens fitting, but everything mentioned here will not necessarily happen in all cases. Different fitters do things in different ways, but there are certain basic functions which all fitters must perform in order to do the job properly.

The preliminary chat

Before starting to examine you the fitter will usually ask you why you want contact lenses and try to decide whether there are likely to be any obvious psychological difficulties or, even, whether you need contact lenses at all! He should also relieve your natural anxiety by explaining what he is going to do and assure you that you are not going to suffer great discomfort when the trial lenses are put on your eyes.

The examination

The next step is for the fitter to check whether or not your eyes are basically healthy, and this applies particularly to the corneas and the conjunctivas. This point can be determined only by careful examination, and for this the fitter uses an ocular microscope. Eye specialists use an instrument called a slit-lamp microscope which enables them to make a most detailed and searching examination of the front part of the eye, in just a few minutes. The better equipped contact lens fitters use the slit-lamp microscope a great deal; others use a simpler form of illuminated magnifier. But it is the skill of the fitter that really matters.

The slit-lamp is a device behind which you sit, with your chin on a shallow cup and your forehead resting against a plastic strap. You will see a bright light and the front lens of the microscope will come to within a couple of inches of your eyes. Don't let this unnerve you.

Next, the fitter must determine the exact prescription required to correct your focusing error, whether it be short sight, long sight and/or astigmatism (see Chapter 2). Sometimes he will do this simply by taking the prescription from your present glasses, using a small optical machine called a focimeter, but this is not really satisfactory as he may not be sure of the accuracy of the glasses. The most careful fitters prefer to test your eyes without any preconceived notions.

The fitter will now check, perhaps by actual measurement, whether your corneas are of unusual size and will note how the lid margins lie in relation to your corneas and whether the corneas are well exposed or largely covered. These factors may influence the decision on what kind of lens may be best for you and, if hard lenses are chosen, whether normal-sized or very small lenses would be best.

Next, the fitter will measure the degree of curvature of your corneas, using an instrument called a keratometer, and you will be asked to put your chin on the rest with your forehead against the strap, in exactly the same way as you did with the slit lamp. In some cases, both instruments may be mounted on the same table and be moved inwards from either side so that you need not move from the central chin rest, between the slit lamp examination and the measuring process known as a keratometry.

The keratometer is a precision instrument which enables the fitter to measure the exact steepness of the curvature of your corneas; it is very likely that your corneas are not evenly curved (as on the surface of a perfect sphere) but have some degree of astigmatism. Usually, the cornea is curved more steeply from top to bottom than from side to side, but this is not always the case. So the fitter will take the measurements on each cornea and it is on these measurements that the selection of the trial contact lenses is based. It is, therefore, essential that the measurements are accurate.

What it feels like

By now you may be feeling a little tense and the fitter will, I hope, offer a few words of comfort and reassure you that having a contact lens on your eye is not the ordeal you may expect. Assuming that the job has been done properly thus far and that the trial lens selected is a reasonably close fit and has been thoroughly cleaned, wetted and placed on your cornea with reasonable skill, you should experience little discomfort and be pleased that you are able to tolerate it so well.

You, as the patient, will help both yourself and the fitter at this stage if you can remain relaxed and trust in his competence. If you are excessively nervous or uncontrolled, you may make it quite impossible for him to proceed any further, either by screwing up your lids or (if the lids are held open) rolling up your eyes, every time he approaches. Of course, no sensible person would deliberately behave like this, and the fact that quite a number do indicates that the reaction is involuntary. Very occasionally – perhaps one in a hundred fittings – the attempt has to be abandoned altogether. On the other hand, many patients are so controlled and apparently unconcerned that I wonder at the power of suggestion. I sometimes even have to tell patients to start blinking after I have put the lens on to the cornea! The most usual response, however, is one of gratified surprise that contact lenses can be so comfortable.

There are very few cases in which nervousness proves to be a major and persistent problem. The eventual realization that a contact lens placed on the eye for the first time is perfectly tolerable, can nearly always overcome the difficulty. In fact, when a well selected lens is properly placed on your eye, it does not actually touch the cornea but rather floats gently on the surface of the tear film. Assuming you don't have too much astigmatism, there will be a continous film of water between the lens and the cornea to act as such an effective cushion that you can tap lightly on the lens with the tip of your finger and you will feel nothing.

Even so, it is undeniable that new lens wearers do experience some discomfort when the lens is first inserted. This is because the lid margins are extremely sensitive and whenever anything touches the surface of the lid edge just behind the lashes, you will automatically jerk your head back.

Now the upper edge of a small contact lens on the cornea will tend to present itself to the margin of the upper lid. Therefore, if you look *up*, or even straight ahead, as soon as the lens is inserted, you may be very aware of the strong sensation as the upper edge of the lens strikes the margin of the lid. If, on the other hand, you look *down*, your upper lid will automatically slip down over the upper edge of the lens and, so long as you keep your eyes in this position, the edge of the lens will not bump against the lid margin. For this reason the contact lens fitter will always ask you to turn your eyes downwards immediately after he has put on the lens. It is this lid sensitivity which makes the main difference in comfort between hard and soft lenses. The latter are so large that the upper lid margin is always below the upper edge of the lens, so the bump is never felt.

While you are maintaining this eyes-down posture you may hardly be aware that you have a lens in your eye. On the other hand you may be aware of a quite strong sensation similar to what you feel when you get an eyelash in your eye. Some people find that the eye waters profusely. It is all a matter of individual sensitivity. If you do find that your eyes water, don't worry. This always stops in a few minutes, as the nerves adapt to the presence of the foreign body. After three or four minutes you will be able to raise your eyes to the straight ahead position without much discomfort, but blinking will still produce a strong sensation and it may be ten to fifteen minutes before you can blink without being very much aware of what you are doing.

The importance of blinking

Because of the sensitivity of the lids, there is a tendency to blink less often than normal; in fact, you will find that you can keep your eyes open between blinks for much longer periods than you usually do. This is *unacceptable*. Quite a lot of contact lens problems arise from unsatisfactory blinking patterns.

A common form of defective blinking is the kind in which the upper lid is lowered just enough to push the lens slightly downward over the cornea, then raised again, so that the lid doesn't have to force its way over the top edge of the lens. This process is much more comfortable than proper blinking and the brain is fooled into thinking that there has been an actual blink. Unfortunately two important things that should have happened, haven't. The first is that the contact lens has not had its regular windscreen wipe and tear film smooth over. So the front surface will soon become dry and cloudy, vision will become very foggy and the proper movement of the upper lid over the lens will become more difficult and uncomfortable. The second thing is more subtle, but is at least as important. It concerns tear film interchange and deserves the full treatment you will find in Chapter 8. To deal with it here would divert us from the real subject of this chapter.

The experience

As soon as you are able to look ahead without your eyes watering, you will begin to appreciate what contact lenses are all about. Wide field of clear vision, pin-sharp clarity, no spots before the eyes, comfortable ears, no misting over when you drink something hot. But to enjoy these advantages permanently there is still quite a way to go and it is by no means certain that the first lenses tried will be the right ones for you. Now the fitter will probably ask you to sit in his waiting room for a while, and you are likely to find yourself taking new interest in your environment.

After you have been wearing the lenses for thirty minutes to one hour, the fitter will call you in again and examine the way the lenses lie on your corneas. This is most easily done with the slit lamp microscope, but some fitters use an illuminated magnifying glass. One of the most important points he will check is how the lenses move when you blink. If he finds, for instance, that the lenses are stuck firmly to the corneas and don't move at all, he will remove the lenses at once, even if you assure him that they are very comfortable. 'Stuck-on' lenses are usually easy to tolerate for the first hour or so but will cause major problems soon after that because of lack of tear film interchange (see Chapter 8). Properly fitting lenses should move and it is important for you to know this, and why.

Importance of lens movement

Lens movement sometimes causes concern to the patient in the early stages of adaptation but, in fact, there would be considerably more cause for concern if the lenses did not move. A well-fitting lens is actually floating on the corneal tear film and is held in place by what we call 'surface tension'. When the curved lens is displaced, this surface tension pulls it back to its central position on the cornea and a satisfactorily fitted lens will do so with a nice springy bounce. So, when the blink starts, the floating lens is first pushed a little downwards by the upper lid, carried further down as the lid closes over it, then carried up high on the cornea by the rising upper lid and, finally, released so that it quickly snaps down to its central position.

A lens that does not behave in this way, when you blink, is probably not satisfactory. At one extreme, a lens that is too steep (with a sharper degree of curvature than the cornea) may not move at all but may act rather like a rubber 'sucker'. At the other, a lens that is too flat, will be extremely mobile and may flop about, with a strong tendency to come off the cornea altogether. At the least, a flat lens will lie low on the cornea and the lower edge may even slip over the edge of the cornea or may rest on the lower lid.

If the fitter is unhappy about the clearance of the lens – as may occur if your cornea is too astigmatic – he may use a harmless yellow dye called fluorescein to stain the tear film and make examination easier. Fluorescein is best applied from sterile, individually packed paper strips. If he uses these the fitter will tear one open and, after moistening the tip with salt solution, will touch the softened end to the tear film behind your lower lid. Either you will feel nothing at all or, at most, a very slight irritation. Now, the fitter will be able to examine your eye with the microscope, also using a rather impressive blue light that causes the fluorescence to glow bright yellow or green. By checking the displaced tear film in this way the fitter can see where it is thick (large clearance) and where it is very thin. Some fitters use fluorescein in every case, others only occasionally and some not at all.

When the lenses have been checked for position and move-ment, you will have a second vision test and it may be that the fitter will put other spectacle lenses in front of the contact lenses to get the best possible clarity. Unless your prescription corres-ponds exactly to the power in his fitting lenses he will add or subtract the extra power to give you perfect vision.

One thing the fitter will be very interested to find out is whether the prescription required with the contact lenses, cor-responds to the prescription needed without them. If you have strong glasses a slight adjustment will have to be made when the prescription is put into contact lenses but, this apart, the power should be the same in both. If the fitter finds that he needs a very different power in the contact lens from that worked out before he put on the contact lens, he will be able to assess whether the lens he is trying is too steep or too flat.

To get everything right, your lens fitter may have to try more than one lens in each eye, perhaps several, because, although he can be very accurate in measuring the curves of your corneas he will still have to choose a trial lens of radius lying somewhere between the flattest and the steepest curves on each cornea. In some cases there may be half a dozen trial lenses available between these two extremes. In addition, he may find that none of the lenses, of a given diameter, within this range, is any good, and he will then have to select a smaller or larger lens.

Don't worry about these changes. You will not have to go through all the initial reactions each time a lens is taken out and a new one inserted. And the necessary changes can be made almost without you feeling anything. For convenience and speed he may use a small plastic sucker to remove the lenses from your corneas and if you just keep your eyes wide open when he is doing this all will be well.

When he has found the lenses that seem best for you, your fitter may suggest a longer period of trial wear or may simply indicate that the fitting is complete and that lenses should now be ordered. A few contact lens fitters actually make their own lenses, but this is now uncommon. The majority obtain lenses from one of a small number of manufacturers who turn out lenses by the million. Some fitters lay in large stocks of lenses and may be able to supply you immediately, but many prefer not to have a lot of stock on hand and order lenses to the specifications determined by the fitting.

Soft lenses

Soft contact lenses are made of a material called hydrogel and, as a considerable proportion of their structure consists of water, they must be kept wet at all times. If a soft lens is allowed to dry, it turns greyish, twists into an irregular shape and becomes hard and brittle. In this condition it is easily broken. When it is re-soaked however, the proper shape is completely restored and the lens becomes very flexible and almost jelly-like.

It has to be said that soft lenses are easier to fit than hard and that one can usually get through the business in a much shorter time. Nevertheless, there are certain basic activities that must never be omitted, whether fitting hard or soft lenses. To begin with, the preliminary microscopic examination of the eyes is essential. Certain conditions, such as infection of the conjunctivas could actually be more dangerous to a person wearing soft lenses than to someone wearing hard, as soft lenses may more easily become contaminated by germs than hard lenses and an infection can be prolonged.

Secondly, the careful determination of the power of lens necessary to correct the focusing error is just as important when fitting soft lenses as when fitting hard. It is especially important for the fitter to know of the presence and degree of any astigmatism, for this may make satisfactory fitting of a soft lens impossible. However, so far as the measurement of the corneal curvature (keratometry) is concerned, this need not be so accurate as when fitting hard lenses, for soft lenses are more tolerant to minor differences in fit.

Assuming your corneas are reasonably spherical, the fitter will select a trial lens which is quite a bit flatter than the cornea. Most soft lenses are larger in diameter than the cornea and some are so big that it is quite a problem to keep the lids wide enough apart to let the lens pass between them. So, having assessed your reactions, he will either just ask you to keep your eyes wide open and look straight ahead, or he may gently hold open your lids. In either case, the important thing is for you to keep looking steadily to the front. It is very frustrating for the fitter if you roll your eyes up every time he tries to pop the lens on to your cornea. With soft lenses you have even less reason to do this than with hard because the degree of immediate comfort is higher. You will probably be surprised how comfortable they are.

If you are nervous, hold on to the idea that a soft contact lens is made of water and held in place by a soft plastic sponge. If you do this you will expect – and experience – very little sensation when the lens is placed on to your eye.

The fitter will then be able to go ahead and examine you on the microscope almost at once. The main things he will be looking at will be the position of the lens – it should sit evenly around the cornea and not hang down – and the amount of movement on blinking. There is really not much more to it than that.

The fitter must, however, check that your vision, with the

lenses, is normal and it may be necessary to add or subtract lens power with additional trial lenses, as in the case of hard lenses, in order to arrive at the final prescription. But because fewer fitting lenses are needed, many practitioners fit from stock and the lenses you try may become your own.

The question of cost

Contrary to what seems to be universally believed, at least in the case of hard lenses it is not simply the lenses you are paying for! The fitting of hard lenses involves skills that can be acquired only after considerable study, training and experience. When you consult a man who possesses this expertise, he commands a fee just as a medical specialist, a solicitor, a financial adviser or any other expert does. The fee will probably also include follow-up check visits.

In the case of soft lenses, the degree of skill needed is less, but the basic cost of the lenses is considerably higher. So, in this case, a larger proportion of what you pay is to cover the cost of the lenses. But no fitter will be qualified to practise if he can fit only soft lenses, so the degree of expertise is just the same.

Also, over the course of a few years, a successful hard lens wearer who takes reasonable care of the lenses, will be likely to pay out a great deal less money than a spectacle-wearing friend. Spectacle frames quickly go out of fashion, get lost or broken and the price of reasonable frames rises constantly. At the present time the cost of a good pair of spectacles is about the same as the cost of fitting and providing a pair of hard lenses. I have seen many patients who have worn the same pair of hard lenses for upwards of ten years and I have often found, on microscopic examination, that the lenses are in almost perfect condition. Certainly, however, one must take into account the cost of soakage solutions and the replacement cost of lost lenses. Much depends on how careful you are. Soft lenses are a much more expensive proposition – probably, in most cases, spectacles are cheaper. This issue is dealt with in Chapter 5.

5

Which Are Best – Hard or Soft?

This is not a question that can be answered in a word, for each kind has much to commend it and a great deal depends on the person who is being fitted. In general, hard lenses are always to be preferred – for the reasons given below – but undeniably, there are patients who seem unable to tolerate hard lenses but who succeed excellently with soft ones.

Occasional wear

The first point to make is that there is no such thing as an 'occasional' hard lens wearer. You either wear hard lenses every day or not at all. The successful hard lens wearer has gradually built up a tolerance until the lenses can be worn all day long; but if, for any reason, they have to be left off for a few days, some of the tolerance will be lost and must be restored by initially resuming wear for a shorter period and progressively increasing the time.

Most soft lenses, on the other hand, can be worn safely, at least for several hours without the wearer having to work up to the required time. Thus it will usually be feasible to use soft lenses for special purposes, such as social or sporting occasions, when glasses are undesirable. Wear, for special social purposes, can, however, be a bit risky as if these activities are unexpectedly prolonged the wearer may forget to remove the lenses before going to bed. This can damage the cornea and result in a painful and even temporarily disabling condition. But, used sensibly, soft contact lenses can be a considerable convenience and anyone who chooses this option could simply wear the lenses every day.

25

Sport

Soft lenses, being larger than hard ones and having better adhesion to the corneas (and to the surrounding conjunctivas), remain more stable on the eyes than hard lenses and are preferred, by some people, for this reason. Those who participate in strenuous sports such as squash may find the additional lens security important. Tennis players may prefer them because there can be special difficulties with hard lenses when serving. Also, the action of looking up can cause hard lenses to drop downwards so that clear vision is lost. In gymnastics, hard lenses may pop out. But it should be said that large numbers of people engage in all sorts of sporting activities, wearing hard lenses, and never have any of these problems.

Psychological problems

Probably the commonest reason for choosing soft rather than hard lenses is the purely psychological one of fear of discomfort. Though the least adequate reason for selecting them, it is a powerful one and probably results in thousands of people wearing soft lenses, when they would be very much better off with hard. Unfortunately, once one has experienced the immediate comfort of soft lenses, one is unlikely to take kindly to the strong sensation experienced when hard lenses are first inserted. As explained in Chapter 4, this sensation soon passes and hard lenses quickly become easily tolerated; but patients who have experienced soft lenses tend to require very strong persuasion to go on persevering when hard lenses are subsequently tried.

Disadvantages of soft lenses

Because the surfaces of soft lenses cannot be cut with the same precision as can hard lenses, and their flexibility carries with it a tendency to bend a little out of the ideal shape, soft lenses can never provide as high a standard of optical performance as hard

26

ones. In some cases, the clarity of central vision will be about as good with soft lenses as with glasses, but it will never be as good as the vision through hard lenses. (The quality of *overall* vision is almost always much better with any kind of contact lenses, than with spectacles.) In patients with astigmatism, the soft lens will simply mould itself to the undesirable curvature of the cornea and the front surface of the lens will then be astigmatic. In such a case the vision with soft lenses will not be nearly as good as is possible with hard. It is true that soft lenses can be obtained with a cylindrical correction for astigmatism, but it is difficult to fit them so that the cylinder lies at the correct axis and they are very expensive.

The question of cost must be considered and there is a good deal more to this than the simple fact that soft lenses cost anything from 50 per cent to 100 per cent more than hard ones. It must also be remembered that whereas hard lenses, properly looked after, last for ever; this is not the case with soft lenses. Carefully tended and cleaned, soft lenses should last for about two years; unfortunately some come to grief after a much shorter time than this and the reasons are as follows.

Careless handling, especially when the lens is not fully wetted, may result in it being torn clean across or an edge being nicked. Ladies with long fingernails must be especially careful not to catch the edge of lenses with the tip of a fingernail as this can be a most expensive activity. Frequent handling, flexing, and just general ageing eventually lead to roughness, cracking and splitting and there is some tendency for soft lenses to lose their elasticity and to become rigid. Sometimes the plastic develops a yellow tint and loses its clarity. Some of these effects can be caused by various eye drops used for medical purposes so it is advisable to remove lenses if eye drops are being used – but particularly if they contain adrenaline.

Another way in which the useful life of a soft lens can be shortened is by protein build-up on the surface. The protein comes from the normal mucus secreted by glands in the conjunctiva and can stick very firmly to the lens. Removal, by special cleaning agents and enzymes (see Chapter 7) is possible but this must be done thoroughly and, in some cases, frequently, if the life of the lens is to be preserved.

Disadvantages of hard lenses

A new hard lens wearer has very little built-in tolerance and should not expect to be able to wear the lenses all day long from the start. A gradual build-up period is necessary and this may take a month or longer. Usually about four hours is the limit to begin with, with an increase in wearing time of 30 minutes to one hour every day. This varies greatly with different patients even if the fit is perfect. Also, if the lenses have to be left off for more than a few days, some of this slowly acquired tolerance will be lost and the wearer will have to be content with a shorter wearing period until full tolerance is again gradually reached. This can be a nuisance and there is a temptation to over-wear the lenses – sometimes with painful results.

Hard lens wearers cannot always achieve morning-to-night tolerance and those who have to remove them before the end of the day often experience an effect called 'spectacle blur'. This is caused by a slight swelling of the corneal epithelium from accumulation of fluid (oedema). If this is localized to the central part of the cornea, it causes a surface bulge and a marked change in focus. Also, the fluid in the tissue causes scattering of light rays, as in a fog, so that vision may be very misty. Spectacle blur suggests that the contact lens fit is not very good. It may clear in a few minutes or may last for hours.

Another similar problem affecting hard lens wearers, is corneal moulding. This can be a major difficulty for the optician who is asked to supply a hard contact lens wearer with glasses, because the focus of the eye is critically affected by the curvature of the cornea and any change in the curvature will markedly alter the focus of the eye. If, for instance, a short-sighted person is wearing hard lenses that are a little too steeply curved on the insides, in a very short time the corneas will push forward in the centres to conform accurately to the hollow in the backs of the lenses and, after being moulded in this way will eventually tend to retain the new shape when the lenses are removed. Such a person will become temporarily more short-sighted and if tested for glasses soon after removing the hard lenses will find the glasses initially satisfactory but too strong some time later, as the corneas revert as they always do to their former shape. If the hard lenses are too flat, the eyes will become temporarily less short-sighted and glasses ordered during that period will be too weak later on. Obviously, hard lenses will not be fitted steep or flat if this can be avoided but it is sometimes necessary to do so to get satisfactory centring and proper movement. Also, in the cases of some patients with astigmatism, corneal moulding may be unavoidable.

Moulding is really only a problem when changing from hard lenses back to spectacles and a successful contact lens wearer will not normally expect to have to do this. While the lenses are being worn, a bit of moulding doesn't do any harm and is certainly not a reason to prefer soft lenses to hard.

Is there anything in between?

New materials are constantly being developed for contact lenses and some combine properties of both hard and soft lenses. The basic ingredients of more than one type of plastic can be mixed together and lenses made from these new blends will usually be softer and more wettable than standard hard lenses made from perspex but may still have some of the tendency to retain shape which is such a desirable property of hard lenses. Most of the mixtures have the additional, major advantage of allowing oxygen to diffuse through. The perfect material is still to be developed, but recent advances have made possible the design of lenses which promise to eliminate some of the disadvantages of both hard and soft lenses (see Chapter 10).

Continuous wear lenses

Great interest has been aroused in recent years in the possibility of contact lenses which can be worn continuously and which need not be removed even at night. Such a possibility did not exist when contact lenses were available only in the hard form and the risks of having them in for longer than the normal day-time wear periods were then extremely high. The problem is, essentially, one of ensuring that the corneal tissues get an adequate supply of oxygen from the atmosphere (see Chapter 8).

With the development of soft lenses of very high water content (manufacturers are now producing lenses in which over 80 per cent of the material is water) and of extreme thinness, oxygen from the atmosphere can penetrate without difficulty to the surface of the cornea. This development is of very great interest to eye doctors, many of whose patients would benefit greatly from the use of contact lenses but who are often too old and shaky, or too concerned at the thought of putting in and taking out lenses, to be able to manage them. In particular, eye surgeons are interested in the use of these continuous wear lenses by patients who have had cataract operations and require thick-lensed, uncomfortably heavy glasses to bring their eyes back into focus again.

Continuous wear lenses are easy to remove and can be taken out by the patient, or by a relative, as a precautionary measure should any concern arise. However, being large and extremely flexible, they are not quite so easy to insert as to remove and, in most cases, the eye specialist would put them in himself.

There are many eye disorders in which very thin, continuous wear contact lenses may be used with great benefit to the patient and these lenses are playing an increasing part in the treatment of many conditions of the front of the eye.

Danger-beware

The question of continuous wear lenses is, of course, also of great interest to the ordinary short-sighted person. But medical opinion is, in this case, not so enthusiastic: there are some dangers and it is questionable whether the minor advantage of not having to remove contact lenses justifies routinely providing patients with these lenses when there is no particular reason to do so. Ultra-thin, high water content, soft lenses are reasonably safe, used on a continual basis, but their widespread use might tempt patients in possession of thicker and lower water content soft lenses, to try to wear *these* for prolonged periods. To do so is to run the risk of suffering a serious complication in which the corneas become water-logged – even wrinkled internally and the vision seriously damaged. The eyes may become intensely congested and the patient suffer severe pain. Under specialist care, the eyes may return to normal in time but the experience is not one which should be risked. Lesser degrees of the same disorder are extremely likely if attempts are made continuously to wear unsuitable contact lenses.

Other important and serious corneal disorders which may arise from the continuous wear of unsuitable lenses are the growth of new blood vessels into the cornea itself with consequent loss of clarity, repeated infection of the eyes from contaminated lenses and a change in the shape of the cornea so that the patient becomes more short-sighted than before.

In addition to problems affecting the wearer, continuous wear of unsuitable lenses tends to cause deposits of protein or fatty material on the surface of the lenses or even a mineralization with a white substance (probably calcium) which becomes incorporated into the lenses. This may occur anything from one month to a year from the onset of wear and, in the former case, makes the cost of wearing contact lenses prohibitive.

Patients with 'continuous-wear' lenses require close supervision. They should be followed up for a minimum of one year. After the lenses are first inserted the patients should be seen at frequent intervals and the lenses removed to allow a microscopic examination of the surface of the corneas. Patients should ideally be seen at intervals of 1 week, 2 weeks, 1 month and then monthly for 1 year. Microscopic examination must be made of the inside of the upper lid as the prolonged wear of contact lenses can cause the lining of the lid to become swollen and develop flat, whitish plaques known as 'cobble stones'.

Another problem that can arise from the continuous wear of contact lenses is the extension into the corneas of tiny branching blood vessels. These indicate that the corneas are not receiving enough oxygen. Blood, of course, carries oxygen and this is the way the body responds when there is a local shortage. Blood vessel invasion of the corneas is a serious matter as this is soon followed by their becoming impervious to light – which may extend far enough inwards to interfere with vision permanently. Once established, these blood vessels will never entirely disappear, although they may in time empty of blood and become 'ghosts'.

My main concern about continuous-wear lenses is that they really do require frequent and skilled supervision, by someone with the proper expertise and equipment. It doesn't take an eye doctor more than a few minutes to check that all is well – and it is in the best interests of people wearing lenses to be examined in this way.

6

How to Insert, Replace and Remove Lenses

This issue often causes the beginner unnecessary worry. In fact, millions of people who now wear contact lenses can look back with amusement at their initial anxieties. It is, of course, the business of the contact lens fitter to help ease the patient through this stage and it is a measure of his skill and experience how well he does so. Once you leave the fitter's consulting room, however, you are on your own and this chapter has been written as a reminder of the various methods you can use and of how to resolve any problem that may arise.

First, I want to remind you of the importance of high standards of cleanliness in any activity connected with contact lenses. Before beginning to insert or remove lenses *wash your hands thoroughly* then carefully rinse off all traces of soap. Secondly, remember when you are inserting, removing or adjusting the position of a lens always to keep both eyes open. If you allow the other eye to shut tightly you will have problems.

Should you accidentally drop a lens on the floor – stand still while you search. A lens can easily be crushed underfoot. Also, if you are washing a lens over a sink, make sure that the plug is in before you start! A slightly tinted lens is much easier to see under water than a clear one; the tint makes no difference to the vision and costs very little extra so it is worth while asking for tinted lenses, preferably grey.

Hard lenses – insertion

The majority of patients have become wholly relaxed about

33

putting on and removing lenses by the time they attend for the first follow-up appointment. Many, at that stage, are able to treat the matter as a joke and refer to their former anxieties with amusement or mild embarrassment. A minority, however, are still having some difficulties and in a small proportion of cases these difficulties may persist – sometimes because the wearer has never had proper instruction.

Putting a contact lens on a cornea is no more difficult than putting it on the tip of your finger but, in practice, there are several factors that can frustrate you. The first is that the eyelids can, and probably will, get in the way long before you can get near the surface of the cornea with your lens. This is a perfectly natural response and is exactly what you have been doing all your life, whenever your eye is threatened. Many experienced contact lens wearers so thoroughly learn to block this impulse that they can keep the eye wide open, without touching the lids, while placing the lens on to the cornea. But very few beginners can expect to perform this feat, so it is necessary, at least at first, to hold the lids open. Because the lid skin is very elastic and just underneath is an important flat muscle which can bring the lid margins together even if the skin is held, the only way to keep them securely apart is to hold them either very near the margins (difficult if the skin is not quite dry) or to secure them by trapping the lashes.

One easy method of holding up the upper lid (which is the larger and more important) is to look right up so that the lashes of the upper lid come to rest just under the bone edge (Figure 4) and then to press the centre of the row of lashes up against the bone with the *middle* finger of your free hand. This gives you extremely effective exposure when you look downwards, as the upper lid is prevented from following the eye down in its normal fashion. All that is necessary now is to pull down the lower lid a little, with a finger placed centrally just below the lid margin, and the whole of the cornea will be widely uncovered. By using the middle finger you leave the index finger free to carry the lens. Note the emphasis on central placement of both restraining fingers: it is no

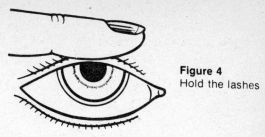

Figure 4
Hold the lashes

good holding the corner of the lid as this will allow the centre to sag across the cornea.

So far so good. You have now learned how to expose the whole of the cornea; but all this effort will be wasted if you turn your eyes to the side or up or down. No matter how effectively you hold your lids apart, you will still be able to get your cornea behind the lid edges so that it will be impossible to get a lens on.

All this may seem too obvious to be worth mentioning, but the reason I do mention it is that, time after time, patients secure their eyelids perfectly then frustrate the whole endeavour by rolling their eyes, usually right upwards, but sometimes to the side. Fortunately, there is an easy way out of this problem. If your lids are properly held and if the contact lens is brought up to the eye on the tip of the index finger, *so that you can look straight into it*, and if you continue to *look straight into it* until it is on your eye, then it can only go on one place – where it should go, right on to the centre of your cornea. If you are *not* looking straight into the lens when applying it to the eye, it will not land on the cornea.

So this is another psychological barrier which has to be overcome, and don't be surprised if you have a bit of difficulty to start with. It goes against all instinct to stare straight at something that is getting nearer and nearer to your eye, with the evident intention of actually touching it! But it is amazing how a reflex habit of a lifetime can be overcome when you find that neither discomfort nor harm is involved.

The method I have suggested of securing the eyelids is probably the best, but some people find it awkward and prefer to hold

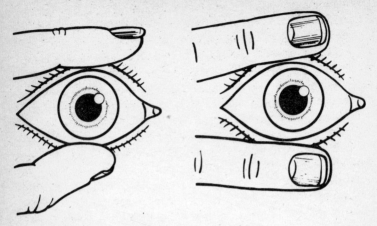

Figure 5 Two methods of holding the lids open.

the lids open with the fingers of one hand (as in Figure 5) while bringing up the lens on a finger of the other hand, because they find it easier to control the finger on which the lens is sitting if that hand is free. It does not matter very much how you do it, so long as you really are keeping the lids wide apart and are keeping the cornea well centred.

One thing you should avoid, however, is holding the lens on a rigid rubber or plastic sucker when putting it on the eye. With such a device you are much more likely to bang the lens painfully against the cornea than if it is resting on the soft pad of your finger. I don't advise using suckers to remove the lenses either, but more about that later in this chapter.

While I am very much in favour of your using a method which enables you to put the contact lens directly on to the cornea, I would not like to suggest that there is no other way of getting the lens there. Some people find it very difficult to place the lens directly on to the cornea and, perhaps because they have found themselves repeatedly rolling the eyes upwards (consequently depositing the lens on the conjunctiva below the cornea), have settled for a method of doing this deliberately and then gently pushing the lens up on to the cornea. This is all right if it is done properly, but remember that the cornea bulges out fairly steeply and the edge of the lens may strike sharply against the start of the corneal curve as you push it up. If you prefer this method, the right way is to pop the lens on to the conjunctiva immediately below the cornea then, by pressing *through the lid*, on to the lower edge of the contact lens, to tilt the upper edge of the lens a little way clear of the eye and then push it up on to the cornea. The whole manoeuvre is done by gentle pressure through the lid.

Incidentally, if you have to move a contact lens which has been displaced from the cornea and is lying on the white of the eye, this is how to do it. Simply feel the lens through the lid, moving your eye in the opposite direction, as necessary. Even if the lens has travelled right up under the upper lid, so that it is barely visible or even completely concealed by the lid, it will be quite easy to slip it forward and down just by looking downwards and gently pushing the lens down with the finger tip placed on the outside of the lid.

Hard lenses – removal

In general, removal is easier than insertion. Lenses are removed, not with the fingers but with the lid margins. When you are wearing lenses your lids, on closing, slip easily over the lens to be in front of it. Indeed, for most of the time your upper lids will be covering the upper part of the front surface of the lenses so that when your eyes close, the lids simply slip down over the front surfaces. If however, your lids are held so wide apart that the lid margins are above and below the edge of the lens, and if the lid margins are then pressed tightly against the cornea, any attempt to bring the lids together will tend to squeeze the contact lens off the cornea.

As when inserting lenses, the cornea must be well centred between the lids or it will not be possible for the lid margins to stay clear of the lens. Once you are sure of this press the lids tightly against the cornea above and below the lens. The most popular way of doing this is to place one or two finger tips on the skin at the outer corner of the eye and pull the skin back and slightly upwards so as to tighten the lids on the cornea. There is a knack in doing this and beginners usually fail because, as soon as they start pulling the skin back, they allow the lids to close over the lens. This makes it impossible for the lens to come out. In the normal course of events, pulling the skin backwards will always bring the lids together and it is essential that you should hold the lids wide (to clear the contact lens) while you are pulling – take care not to pull very hard!

Gently pull the lids back and a little upwards. If, while maintaining the lid margins tight against the cornea, you now try to blink, or turn your eye towards your nose, the tight lid margins will catch the edges of the lens and pop it out of your eye into the palm of your other hand, held conveniently close to receive it. This is probably the best method, especially for the younger wearer, whose lids are normally reasonably tight.

Older people's lids are often quite lax and the edges may turn out slightly making it difficult or impossible to use this method. In this case, keep the lid margins against the cornea by pressing them directly on with the finger tips then bring them together to catch on the upper and lower margins of the lens and pop it out.

In using either of these methods the lens will often stick to the lashes and you may wonder what has happened to it. The expert will always succeed in dropping the lens into her hand, but until you acquire this degree of skill, do your lens removing over a flat surface on which you have spread a clean towel.

Solid plastic sucker

This is a device which I view with mixed feelings, having once or twice seen damage resulting from the unskilled application of one of these devices to the naked cornea. It is a non-squeezable gadget with a very thin-cupped business end, which grips the lens strongly. I don't think it is possible to do any very serious harm, but there is no doubt that you can give yourself a very sore eye if you are careless. The sucker is a most efficient way of removing a hard contact lens. Unfortunately, if you happen not to have a lens on the cornea, it will grip the corneal epithelium instead, with very painful results. You will be incapacitated for a couple of days and will not be able to wear contact lenses for about three weeks.

If you should get a plastic remover stuck on to your cornea, on no account try to pull it off. Instead, try gently to slide it across to the edge of the cornea and free it as it passes on to the conjunctiva. Even if it retains its adhesion, you will do no harm by pulling it straight off the conjunctiva.

A much safer, although less efficient, type of lens remover is the hollow, compressible, type made of rubber or plastic. There is little chance of doing yourself an injury with this type of device, as you can always release it, quite easily, by squeezing. Unfortunately, however, the grip is insecure unless the device is in good condition, the contact lens properly wetted and the timing of the squeeze and release just right. The sucker is handy for removing a lens that has slipped off the cornea and become stuck on the conjunctiva, especially if it is high up behind the upper lid and cannot be eased down. But in this case it is advisable to seek the help of someone else while you turn your eye as hard as you can in the direction opposite to where the lens is sitting (turn your head up and look down).

People with arthritis, or who are very clumsy with their fingers, may consider snipping off the closed end of one of these suckers and pushing the opening thus made over the end of a short length of solid glass rod of suitable diameter. Enough of the sucker should be left free to allow squeezing. Such a device may be found useful in inserting and removing lenses. The secret is to have a source of light behind the far end of the rod, so that the contact lens wearer can sight down through the centre of the lens and the glass rod and thus ensure proper alignment. But take great care to avoid bumping the lens on the cornea – the finger tip is always preferable.

Soft lenses – insertion

Although soft lenses are considerably larger than hard lenses they are almost as easy to insert. If you can hold your lids wide enough apart, you can use the method described above for the insertion of hard lenses and you will find that the lens nestles on to your cornea with no trouble at all and with almost no sensation. There is, however, an annoying tendency for the lens to touch the lid margin or the lashes at the moment of insertion and to be knocked off the finger tip. For this reason, many soft lens wearers adopt the slightly different method described below.

Having balanced the lens on your fore-finger tip, pull the margin of the lower lid well down with your second finger tip and look upwards so that a good area of the white of your eye is exposed. This part of the eye is quite insensitive and can be touched without pain or discomfort, and you will find it easy to let the lens fall directly on to it. Because the soft lens is so large, the upper half will flop on to the lower part of the cornea and if you now look directly to the front the lens will slip upwards until it is centred on the cornea. If there is any tendency for the lens to refuse to move up on to the cornea, simply keep the tip of your finger on it while you look straight ahead. This will ensure that the lens is properly centred and when you take your finger away it will remain so.

Soft lenses, especially the ultra-thin type, are rather floppy when first taken from their soakage solution. It is, therefore, sometimes advantageous to wait for a minute or two to allow each lens to become slightly more rigid before applying it to the cornea. Don't wait too long or the lens will become quite hard and will begin to distort so that you will have to wet it again before attempting insertion.

Soft lenses – removal

This is very easy. Start by getting accustomed to touching the front of the lens while it is on your eye, and do this several times until you have overcome your nervousness. The lens acts as a kind of cushion so you will feel practically nothing. It is important, when you are doing this, not to allow your eye to roll upwards or to the side as this may carry the lens off the cornea. When you are able, quite happily, to look straight ahead with wide open lids while touching the centre of the contact lens, you are in a good position to remove the lens.

Slide the lens downwards on to the white of the eye below the cornea simply by placing the tip of your finger on the centre of the lens and then looking upwards – really, the reverse of the last part of the method described for putting the soft lens on the cornea. Once the contact lens is down on to the conjunctiva you will find it the simplest thing in the world to pinch it off the eye using the tips of the thumb and first finger. If your fingertips tend to slip on the lens, just dry them thoroughly and you will have no further problems.

It isn't really necessary to slide the lens off the cornea before pinching it off the eye and many people pinch them directly off the cornea. But if you do this, be careful to ensure that the edges of your fingernails are turned well outwards so that there is no possibility of scratching the cornea. If your fingernails are very long avoid the pinching method altogether, or cut your nails to a safer, shorter length.

If you prefer to keep long fingernails, it is still possible to remove soft lenses safely but either you must wear rubber gloves or finger stalls, or resort to the method described for hard lenses in which the lid margins are pressed tightly against the eye above and below the lens and are then brought together to squeeze it off the cornea. Some people actually succeed in doing this by the standard hard lens method of pulling the skin back and up at the outer angle of the eye.

But because soft lenses are much larger than hard lenses and are more closely applied to the eye, it is difficult to ensure that the lid margins press on the white above and below the upper and lower edge of the lens and don't just press the lens even more firmly on to the cornea. The tendency for the lids to do this is quite strong and you might well find that you are just not getting anywhere. If this is so, you would be better to fall back on the second method, placing the tips of your first or second fingers of both hands on the lid margins, and using your fingers to press the lids against your eye and squeeze off the lens. If you use this method, don't put the fingertips back from the margins of the lids. If you *do*, the margins will roll outwards and not catch the edge of the lens. Also, be careful to place your fingertips exactly in the centres of the lid margins and not to the side and look directly ahead when you start squeezing.

All this takes much longer to describe than to do and once you have the knack you will wonder what all the fuss was about.

Problems of post-cataract patients

Sometimes the people who need contact lenses most are those who may have the greatest difficulty in inserting and removing them. I touch on the question of contact lenses for people who have had cataract surgery in Chapter 9, but this seems a good place to deal with some of the problems such people have in inserting lenses, and how these may be relieved. In the first place, a patient who has had a cataract removed has a very long-sighted eye so that the nearer an object is brought, the more blurred it becomes. Post-cataract patients should therefore always have glasses, whether or not they wear contact lenses, and the reading glasses should be worn while everything is being made ready for the insertion of the contact lenses. Shakiness and poor co-ordination mean that lenses will often be dropped, so a towel should be spread out.

It is sometimes useful to have a spectacle frame modified, with one lens only, and with the lower part of the frame that is empty cut away. When one contact lens has been inserted through the empty half, the frame is removed and the other contact lens put in. Many post-cataract patients learn to insert lenses by touch alone; the best way for them to control the lids is the standard hard lens method described above as this helps to steady the finger bearing the lens. Some have found the sucker on the glass rod idea helpful. A magnifying shaving mirror can be a valuable – even indispensable – aid.

Such patients are usually old and the lid margins lax and sometimes turned outwards, so that the conventional skin-pulling method of contact lens removal often fails. The method in which the lid margins are pressed on to the eye with the finger tips is more likely to succeed, but this, too, is more difficult in old people than in young. Careful and informed use of squeeze-type rubber suckers may be a great help to such patients but the solid plastic type should *never* be risked. There is one tip which should be remembered when real difficulty is encountered. An ordinary eye bath full of salt water (1 teaspoon of salt to 1 pint of water) may be used to float the lens out of the eye. The full bath is applied to the eye, as the patient bends forward, and a few blinks under water will invariably do the trick.

Soft lenses can always be pinched off so long as the fingers are dry.

7

Care of Lenses

The advice given in this chapter could make the difference between long-term success and a pair of contact lenses abandoned and left, sadly, in a dressing-table drawer.

The first thing to remember is that everything in our environment, including our skin, is to some degree contaminated by germs. Even in an operating theatre only certain designated areas are free from infecting organisms, and in everyday life we can never hope to achieve the high degree of sterility required for surgery. Fortunately, this is unnecessary, as the defence mechanisms of the body can readily cope with the odd organism.

What we are trying to avoid is gross contamination which will overcome the normal body resistance. Such contamination is, unfortunately, only too common so we must assume that heavy contamination is to be found on any surface or object which might have been touched, coughed or sneezed over or indeed had any contact, direct or indirect, with any person. I am not suggesting that the contact lens wearer need be obsessive but simply that he or she should be aware that unwashed hands do carry potentially harmful organisms which can be easily picked up from bus and tube hangers, library books, supermarket trolleys and the door handles of public and private toilets, or anything else people commonly touch. The moral of all this is that *before you touch your contact lenses, or even their containers, you should wash your hands*.

Storage and cleaning of hard lenses

Some people carefully dry their contact lenses after removing them and store them in plastic lined metal containers with two compartments. There are a number of objections to this, not the least of which is that repeated drying of lenses leads to an accumulation of fine scratches on the surfaces of the lenses so that they end up looking like ground glass. Not only does this reduce the clarity of vision, is also greatly increases the chances of infection (germs can collect in the scratches) and makes the lenses uncomfortable. I have seen severe intolerance to arise solely as a result of heavily scratched lenses.

The second objection to dry storage is that one is forced to go through quite a lengthy process of cleaning and re-wetting the lenses each time they are put in. Standard hard lens material does not wet easily and it is common for such dry stored lenses to be put on to the corneas with a small area of the lens not completely wetted. A dry spot causes discomfort and may even lead to a corneal abrasion. The only advantage of dry storage that I am aware of, is that one is spared the risk from contaminated soakage solutions.

For very good reasons, the great majority of hard lens wearers adopt the wet-storage option and use one of the variety of double – ended or double-compartment, screw-capped, water-tight containers in which the lenses rest in a soakage fluid when not being worn. Thus, the lenses are never allowed to dry, and maintain their surfaces in a permanently clean state.

The soakage solutions contain a mild antiseptic (often a mercurial compound such as Thiomersal) which should deal effectively with most micro-organisms present in reasonably small numbers, so long as the solution is changed and the case thoroughly cleaned about once a week. The effectiveness of the solution depends also on the degree of contamination of the lenses by organic matter coming from the glands in the conjunctiva and in the lids. Some people produce more mucus and sebaceous secretion than others, especially during the early stages of wearing contact lenses. All traces of this, together with any dried salt, should be carefully cleaned off the lenses as described below, before they are put into the soakage solution.

45

Routine cleaning

Put the lens on the palm of your hand, hollow side up and fill the hollow with lens cleaning solution. Then, with the tip of a finger of the other hand, rub the solution carefully but thoroughly on to both surfaces of the lens for about half a minute. Then, take the lens by its edge (do not touch the inside after the initial cleaning) and rinse it thoroughly under a running tap: *always see that the plug is in* before doing this. The lens should now be inspected to see if any dry or greasy spots remain. This is best done by holding the lens up to a light and looking through it. If any dry spots are seen, the whole process should be repeated.

In spite of conscientious cleaning by this method, lenses may from time to time become more heavily contaminated or may come in contact with grease, cosmetics, nail polish etc. In this case, you may have to use something stronger but be very careful – Perspex (PMMA) lenses can be destroyed by unsuitable solvents such as alcohol, acetone, petrol or ether. Ordinary household washing-up liquid is safe, or you may try a little culinary vinegar, carbon tetrachloride or calamine lotion. Any such liquid must be carefully washed off the lens before it is put into the soaking solution in its container. If a solvent is used, remove it with a detergent and in turn, wash this off with water and put the lens in soaking solution before wearing it again.

You may be tempted to supplement your cleaning by the use of a tissue – don't! Tissue fibres will scratch the lenses.

Solutions

The variety of contact lens solutions available can confuse the beginner who may feel that some dreadful calamity will attend the use of the wrong one. In fact, very little harm will arise as long as hard and soft lens solutions are not confused, and a clear distinction is made between wetting/soaking solutions, on the one hand, and cleaning solutions on the other. Wetting and soaking solutions should be harmless to the eye, but cleaning solutions must always be carefully washed off the lenses before they are worn. Cleaning solutions generally contain a fairly strong detergent and if you put on a lens without thoroughly rinsing this off you will be in no doubt as to your mistake!

Wetting solutions

The surface of a dry PMMA lens tends to repel water and is difficult to wet. This is a major disadvantage as it is essential that the lens should be completely wet before it is inserted. (I once had a patient who persisted in putting dry lenses into her eyes and could not understand why they were so much less comfortable than when I fitted them!) Fortunately, there are compounds known as wetting agents which spread easily over surfaces such as PMMA and link easily with water. One such agent, commonly used, is polyvinyl alcohol and many wetting solutions contain this.

Soaking solutions

The purpose of these is to keep the lens wet between periods of wear, to keep bacteria at bay and to help in cleaning the lens. Because of this, such solutions invariably contain an antiseptic such as Thiomersal or benzalkonium chloride and usually some kind of wetting agent.

Combined solutions

It is probably unnecessary to separate the functions of wetting and storing. Certainly, many patients get by very satisfactorily with one solution for cleaning and another for wetting and storage. Please note that saliva is *not* a suitable wetting or cleaning solution. It is quite an effective wetting agent but it can also be an effective source of germs and if you use saliva constantly it is only a matter of time before you get an eye infection. Saliva contains a host of potentially harmful bacteria, and, in about 5 per cent of the population, a particular nasty called pseudomonas aeruginosa which is the eye doctor's nightmare.

Storage and cleaning of soft lenses

This is somewhat more complicated than with hard lenses and is another cogent reason why hard lenses are to be preferred. Soft lenses are both more easily contaminated than hard and more difficult to keep clean and to sterilize. You can easily sterilize a soft lens by boiling (I am referring here to conventional soft lenses of less than 60 per cent water content – which may be safely boiled) but if you do this without first cleaning off any protein deposits, you will seal the protein into the lens and eventually ruin it.

If, on the other hand, you avoid boiling and use antiseptic soakage solutions, these will be present in the lens when you wear it and you may suffer chemical damage to your cornea. It has been estimated that about one third of all soft contact lens wearers who use chemical disinfectant develop a reaction to these compounds. One commonly used antiseptic agent, benzalkonium chloride has been shown to concentrate in soft lenses and to be an occasional cause of quite severe corneal damage. Indeed many of the preservatives used in hard lens solutions do this and that is the main reason why hard lens solutions should not be used with soft lenses. Even Thiomersal, which has long been considered a safe preservative for soft lens solutions has now been shown to be capable of producing a chronic inflammation of the conjunctivas, with new vessel growth into the corneas, after many months of use.

As you will see, there is a good deal to be said for sterilizing soft lenses by boiling and a variety of small, automatic boiling units are available. Some do not actually reach boiling point but are thermostatically controlled to keep the temperature at about 80°C for about 10 minutes or so. This will kill most organisms. But there are snags with boiling too. The main one, as already mentioned, is that before doing so, the lenses must be carefully cleaned of all foreign material. This can be done in several ways. The best, at present, is to use enzyme cleaners which break down the protein deposits and free them from the lenses. The enzymes do not affect the lenses and are obtainable in the form of tablets which are dissolved in distilled water in a suitable container and the contact lenses soaked in the solution for at least two hours. Lenses may safely be left in the solution overnight. Enzyme cleaning should be done once a week if you boil your lenses but may be required only once a month if you use chemical disinfecting solutions.

If you boil lenses use distilled rather than tap water, to avoid getting your lenses furred. Another snag is that boilers occasionally go dry, with disastrous effects on your lenses.

In spite of the risks and disadvantages, the majority of soft lens wearers rely on antiseptic soakage solutions and the majority seem to get away with it. New disinfecting substances are constantly being tried – manufacturers are by no means complacent about the number of patients who develop red, itchy, burning eyes as a result of sensitivity to the chemicals used in soakage solutions.

Containers

The variety of these is considerable and the designs have, in general, improved. Leakage of solution should now be a thing of the past so long as containers are discarded before deterioration of materials occurs. When lenses – especially soft lenses – are being put away, great care should be exercised to ensure that the lens is well within the body of the container and does not become trapped in the threads of the screw cap. Once within the fluid, untinted lenses are invisible and accidents can happen. Hard lenses can, and should, be slightly tinted (see page 66) but this is less common with soft lenses – so extra care is required. I suppose nearly every new wearer goes through the panic reaction of thinking that the lenses have been lost, when, in fact, they are nestling happily at the bottom of the container. It is worth mentioning in this context, that a soft lens may sometimes drape itself so closely and inconspicuously around the tip of a finger as to give rise to the conviction that it has been lost. So, if a lens seems, incomprehensibly, to disappear, check your fingertips!

The most important thing to say about containers is that they are liable to get very dirty and should be thoroughly washed, even scrubbed out with a toothbrush, from time to time. It is easy to forget that, although you may be scrupulous in keeping your lenses clean, they may be contaminated every time they are stored in the container.

8

Lens Tolerance and Adaptation

When you first put a hard contact lens on your cornea, you will experience fairly severe intolerance caused mainly by the very thought of having something in your eye, but also by the sensitivity of the upper lid margin. These factors often lead to watering and, sometimes, a strong impulse to squeeze your lids tightly together. But I have hardly ever had a patient who continued to experience this reaction for more than five or ten minutes, assuming the fit of the lens is reasonable. In almost all cases the watering quickly stops and the eyelid muscles relax. When this happens you will probably think that you have got over the problem and may be surprised and disappointed to find that when you try the lenses again the next day, the same things happen all over again. But these affects are never quite so severe on the second occasion as on the first, and tend to last for a shorter time. Indeed, within a few days they will probably be so mild as to be almost unnoticeable. Most contact lens wearers soon forget all about them.

But there is another sense in which we have to consider tolerance; and that is the tolerance of your corneas to being kept short of oxygen – oxygen is the one vital element without which living tissues soon cease to live. Normally, the tissues of the body are supplied with oxygen which enters through the lungs and is transported everywhere via the red blood corpuscles. This is one of the main functions of the blood and the reason why almost all the structures of the body contain a vast network of small branching blood vessels. The corneas, however, are transparent and cannot have arteries and veins running into them, so they get their oxygen direct from the air by diffusion through the

51

tear film on the corneal surface.

A contact lens tightly sealed on to a cornea would seriously interfere with this access of oxygen, so we have to be sure that either the lens allows oxygen to pass through it or that it moves about freely enough to let oxygen in behind it. In fact, oxygen from the air dissolves in the tear film on the cornea and, so long as freshly oxygenated tear fluid can mix freely with the layer of tears behind the lens, all will be well. It is the fitter's duty to ensure, in the case of PMMA hard lenses – which are completely impermeable to oxygen – that this is so.

But even if all is as it should be, your corneas will still be getting less oxygen than normal and may, at first, protest. It is simple common sense therefore, to ensure that the change from full oxygen access to restricted access should be made gradually so that the corneas can adapt to the new conditions.

For this reason your fitter will always provide you with a wearing schedule to cover the first few weeks of hard lens wear. It is very important that you should adhere to this scheme of gradually building up the wearing time and that you should not run ahead of the system. Most schedules will be pretty conservative and most hard contact lens wearers could possibly get away with wearing their lenses for longer periods than recommended during the adaptation period. But to do so is to run the risk of damaging the outer surface of the corneas which, although not usually serious in the long term, could put you off contact lenses for life. Alternatively, surface damage could lead to a condition greatly reducing your tolerance to hard contact lenses or even make them impossible to tolerate altogether.

The cells forming the epithelial layer actually die if the oxygen supply is cut off, or reduced to too low a level. The death of the epithelium occurs only over the central part of the cornea, because the cells near the edge can get oxygen from the network of small blood vessels in the tissues around the transparent part. These surviving epithelial cells are the source of a new cover for the bare central area, but before they provide this the person with the corneal 'abrasion' (as it is often inaccurately named) suffers whenever the lids slide over the exposed central area. This is because the corneal nerves, instead of being protected by the epithelium, are now exposed to direct stimulation by anything that rubs against them. Even the gentle movement of the smooth inner surface of the upper lid is extremely painful. The result is that the patient is forced to resort to keeping the damaged eye or eyes closed and is thus, temporarily, severely disabled. There is also considerable reflex watering of the eyes and the tight squeezing of the lids may be so strong as to prevent the tears from passing out, until the patient is finally persuaded to relax.

But it is very seldom that a patient has to tolerate this kind of distress for more than a few hours: renewal of the epithelium is so rapid that relief is soon obtained. Doctors sometimes treat this condition with local anaesthetic drops but, while these afford rapid relief of pain they are toxic to the remaining edge cells and can prevent normal recovery. Cases have been reported of local anaesthetic drops, used in this condition, leading to so much cell damage that corneal ulceration and even perforation has resulted. Local anaesthetic drops should *never* be used in this condition.

The proper treatment is to prevent infection with antibiotic drops and to let nature do the rest, keeping the eyes shut for as long as the pain persists. The great majority of cases will recover fully without any treatment at all, apart from keeping the eyes shut.

I hope that the above description of oxygen-lack epithelial loss will be enough to discourage you from forging ahead of your initial wearing schedule or from over-wearing hard contact lenses when you are well adapted.

There is, however, one golden rule to be observed if you want to avoid this kind of trouble completely. It is based on the fact that, long before it dies, the corneal epithelium becomes swollen and soggy from the accumulation of fluid and develops a fogginess or 'veiling' which will almost always be noticeable to the wearer. This is usually associated with renewed discomfort. The rule is that one should never go on wearing contact lenses after the vision has become even slightly fogged. If you immediately take out the lenses at this early stage, the corneal epithelia will soon return to normal and you will not suffer the misfortune described above.

It is interesting and important to note that epithelial death from oxygen lack actually occurs most commonly, not during the early adaptation period but in hard contact lens wearers who have become completely and successfully adapted to all-day wear. Such a person may, for a variety of reasons, decide to leave in the lenses for several hours longer than usual. During this time he may experience discomfort and notice that the vision has become a bit foggy. If he ignores this the discomfort will often pass away and the wearer may think that everything is all right. In fact, his corneal nerves have become blunted with prolonged stimulation, and when he takes off his lenses, stripping off the dead epithelium with them, he may still not feel much discomfort initially. But a few hours later, when the corneal nerves have recovered the pain will begin.

Soft lenses

The position with soft lenses is slightly different and, in some ways, more dangerous. The main reason why soft lenses can safely be worn for longer periods than hard lenses and why tolerance is built up more quickly, is that a quantity of oxygen can diffuse through the lens by being dissolved in the water which partly constitutes the lens. This is especially true of ultra-thin, high water content lenses, many of which offer so little resistance to the passage of oxygen that over-wear is almost impossible. Unfortunately, many soft lens wearers have no idea of whether their lenses are thick or thin, high or low water content or of what material they are made. Thus, there is a risk to those whose soft lenses are not suitable for extended wear. This risk is further increased by the very factor that makes soft lenses so popular – the high degree of comfort. Even after corneal epithelial death has occurred soft lenses may act as 'bandages' and prevent symptoms from being experienced. They will not, however, conceal the fogging of vision arising from epithelial oedema, so the person concerned is likely to be alerted to what is happening and at once remove the lenses.

So, once again, the moral is – know the limits of your tolerance and try to stay within them but, if you do extend the period, look out for fogging – which is the indication that lenses should be removed *at once*.

Problems with lenses

This section is concerned with problems arising after you have been satisfactorily fitted and have overcome the initial stages of discomfort. Any problems arising during the first two or three weeks after receiving your lenses are very much the business of your fitter, and should certainly be referred to him as they may arise either from inadequacies in the fit of the lenses or from your failing to understand, or to follow, the instructions and advice you have been given. In either event, it is the fitter's responsibility to put things right. It should not be difficult for him to discover, by careful questioning and examination, exactly what is wrong.

Symptoms, such as a tendency to watering or mild discomfort, which are simply due to your not yet having achieved adaptation, will always improve with time. Those which get worse with time are not adaptive, and must be attended to. These include blurred or foggy vision, severe discomfort and watering, irritation or redness of the eyes. If you experience any of these problems leave off your lenses or, at the very least, cut down considerably on the length of time you wear them, and report the trouble without delay.

Foggy vision
If this occurs as soon as you put in your lenses you should suspect that they have not been properly cleaned and should remove

them and clean them thoroughly. Another cause is inadequate blinking, so that the front surfaces of the lenses become dry. Poor blinking is an important cause of trouble and you should be quite sure that you are closing your eyes properly each time: it is very easy to think that you are blinking when, in fact, you are merely tapping your upper lid margin on the top of the lens and shifting it slightly.

Watch out for fogginess of vision coming on after two or three hours of lens wear. If this happens you must consider the possibility that your corneas are not getting enough oxygen and the fogginess is the result of oedema. This is almost certainly the case if the fogginess persistently comes on after a fixed period of wear and does not clear until after the lenses have been removed. Some minor fogginess is quite common during adaptation but persistent fogging is always unacceptable and must be reported.

Corneal oedema may settle as your corneas adapt but, if you suspect that it is present do *not* extend the period of wear unless and until the fogginess has stopped occurring.

Spectacle blur

This is often connected with corneal oedema and is a mistiness or blurring of vision experienced after the contact lenses are removed and the glasses resumed. It may last only half an hour or so, or may persist for hours.

Another cause of spectacle blur is moulding of the corneas by lenses which are flatter or steeper than the corneas. These temporary changes in the curvature of the corneas will change the focus of the eyes so that the refractive error may be made worse or better. In myopia, flattening of the corneas will improve the uncorrected vision. Marked spectacle blur should certainly be reported. It is not necessarily serious, but is often an indication that the fit of the lenses is not perfect.

Loss of visual clarity with lenses

By this I mean that the vision is out of focus rather than foggy. The first thing to consider (assuming your lenses are of different power) is that you have accidentally switched right for left. This is easily checked. Another cause is the slight excess of watering common in the early stage of adaptation. This will rapidly lessen and will almost always settle within a few days. Persistent watering indicates that something is wrong. Consult your fitter.

A more serious cause, and one that may require the lenses to be changed, is poor centring so that you are looking partly through the optical zone of the lens and partly through the edge. In some cases, centring improves with time but it usually indicates that the fit is inadequate. In this condition, vision will usually clear temporarily when you blink, but quickly revert to the blurring.

Sometimes loss of clarity is caused by a lens becoming accidentally warped, perhaps by being put into the container carelessly, Very occasionally, a contact lens wearer may have had a change in the refraction, so that the power of the contact lenses is no longer appropriate. This, however, is quite uncommon.

Pain

Acute pain occurring immediately after putting in lenses can be due to two main causes – either you have scratched the cornea with the edge of the lens or a piece of grit has found its way underneath. This should never happen if your hygiene is good. In either case, the lenses should be removed. If you still feel pain on blinking, you probably have a corneal injury and you should leave off your lenses and seek advice. But if your eye now feels completely comfortable, clean the lenses carefully and try again.

Corneal abrasion

I have already touched on this, but the condition is so common and alarming that a full account is justified.

The term is misleading as the commonest cause in contact lens wearers has nothing to do with rubbing or abrading the cornea. Rather it is the result of overwear of lenses so that the central part of the corneal epithelium suffers oxygen deprivation of such degree that the cells die. The oedema, which is the first stage of the process, is completely painless, but vision will almost certainly be fogged and this is a warning sign. Characteristically, the acute symptoms: strong foreign body sensation made worse by blinking, severe spasm of the muscle surrounding the eyes, severe watering, pain and redness – come on some hours after the lenses have been removed, often when the patient is sleeping, so that he wakes in considerable distress.

The usual preliminary to corneal abrasion is that the patient has adapted well to lenses but after leaving them off for a period of days or weeks, has resumed wear and, instead of building up tolerance gradually has worn them for the normal time, or even longer. If you have this experience, the most important thing is to realize what has happened and to avoid panic. Don't try to keep your eyes open; gently closed lids offer the best cover for the bare and sensitive corneas and you may find it comforting to keep pads (dry or moist, as you prefer) on your closed lids. Pads are best secured with two strips of sticky tape stretched from the centre of the forehead to the cheek. If you cannot obtain standard eye-pads, use folded sterile gauze, lint or cotton wool.

The epithelium will heal in about a day and you will then be more comfortable, but you should seek medical advice as soon as you can and it is desirable that you should have antibiotic drops (such as Chloromycetin) three or four times a day to prevent the abrasion from becoming infected. Contact lenses should be left off for three weeks after the abrasion has healed and then you must build up your tolerance again as gradually as if you were a first time wearer.

Excessive sensitivity to lenses

A successful wearer is unlikely, at first, to be able completely to forget that lenses are being worn, but should certainly not be constantly and uncomfortably aware of their presence and, as adaptation improves, the periods of almost total unawareness should lengthen. Many people develop a surprising degree of tolerance. I remember a young barrister who, having thought he had lost one contact lens, drove from Edinburgh to London with two lenses in the same eye!

If awareness is, from the beginning, much greater in one eye than in the other, this suggests that the lens in one eye was not properly fitted. But if, after a long period of satisfactory comfort, constant awareness develops in one eye, this suggests that a lens has become either scratched or contaminated with dried mucus or salt, or the edge nicked. If careful examination with a strong magnifier reveals defects of this kind, the remedy is a replacement lens.

A great many instances of excessive awareness of contact lenses are simply due to a decrease in the standard of care and cleanliness of lenses which, in time become greasy, poorly wetted, dirty, contaminated, scratched or even cracked.

Late intolerance

This is a very distressing condition which affects people who have been wearing contact lenses with complete satisfaction and comfort, often for years, and who then, for no apparent reason, find that their degree of tolerance begins to diminish and periods of comfortable wear become progressively shorter. Usually, the people concerned have been accustomed to all-day wear with no problems at all. The cause of this quite common misfortune is obscure but it is probably connected with oxygen supply to the corneal epithelium. Happily, the majority of people who suffer this experience can be restored to comfortable all-day wear by a change, not in the design or fit of the lenses, but in a change of the material from which the lenses are made – possibly to Cellulose acetate butyrate (CAB) or some other gas-permeable material.

Photophobia

This sounds rather ominous, but simply means an undue degree of sensitivity to light. This is almost universal in people beginning to wear contact lenses. It tends to be rather worse with hard lenses than with soft ones. The trouble is probably partly due to the concentration of light in the pupil and partly to the slight irritation to the corneal nerves by the presence of the lens. It is often severe enough to force new contact lens wearers to put on sunglasses, but can be expected, in almost all cases, to disappear in time. A mild tint in the lenses may help to minimize the problem and incidentally is quite a good idea, as a tinted lens is easier to find when dropped in water or when in soakage solution.

9

Special Cases and Applications

Apart from their normal function in the correction of short and long sight, contact lenses have a great deal to offer various other kinds of people. For many of these, contact lenses may be a great deal more important than they are to people with simple refractive errors who can, if they wish, wear glasses. So I would like to say something about these special cases.

Aphakia

For many years, patients who have had cataract surgery (ie who have had their internal eye lenses removed and who have not, for various reasons, been given lens implants) have been disappointed, initially, with the quality of the vision using conventional glasses. The lenses in these glasses have to be so strong and thick that, although vision through the centre of the lenses can be quite clear and sharp, the view round about becomes progressively more distorted, as the patients look sideways, until the image through the edges of the spectacle lenses disappears altogether. In addition, spectacles cause about a 30 per cent enlargement of the image seen, so that objects appear to be nearer than they are and dangers consequently arise in handling domestic equipment.

The improvement in vision enjoyed by these people when they change from spectacles to contact lenses is truly remarkable and in the past many of them have been gravely disappointed when they found they could not manage the handling of hard lenses.

The reason that contact lenses are so much more satisfactory than glasses in these cases is that not only do the lenses more efficiently correct the severe focusing error of the eyes but they

61

also move with the eyes so that the patient is always looking through the centre of the lens.

Patients are usually astonished when first they experience the quality of vision with contact lenses, as compared with their glasses. Instead of a narrow, severely restricted field of clear vision, leading to great difficulty in walking downstairs and severe anxiety in crossing roads, these patients are restored to a quality and breadth of vision such as many of them have not experienced for years. The power of the lenses is calculated for distant viewing and ordinary low-power reading glasses are worn on top of the contact lenses for reading. Contact lenses have much to offer these patients, unless they are very frail or, for other reasons, completely unable to manage them.

Obviously there are problems. I have found that many patients I have operated upon for cataract, and who would benefit markedly from contact lenses, are nervous at the thought of them. In many cases, I have felt justified in putting on a hard contact lens, without preliminary warning, simply to give the patient an opportunity to see how marvellously the vision can be improved. I have seldom been disappointed with the response. I have had many patients who had become depressed and tearful over the difficulties of coping with spectacles after cataract surgery, and whose whole outlook has been changed by the experience of contact lenses.

Many such patients tell me that they are barely aware of the sensation of the lens, even from the moment of insertion. This ready acceptance, however, is another encouragement to over-wear.

The real drawback in the case of aphakic patients, is that most of them are old, many are shaky and for these and other reasons, may have difficulty in inserting and removing lenses. I have tried to offer as much help as I can, on this point, in Chapter 6, but many of these people have to rely on the assistance of a member of the family. It is especially in such cases that the continuous wear contact lens, used under the close supervision of an eye specialist, comes into its own, and it is this that I feel to be the main justification for such supervision.

Congenital cataracts

Aphakia is not confined to the old. Babies born with dense cataracts (congenital cataracts) must be operated upon at a very early age – within a few weeks of birth – and the lenses removed, if there is to be any hope of reasonable vision in later life. Not only must the opaque lenses be removed, but the vision must immediately be brought into focus by some effective means, and there is, at present, no way to do this except with contact lenses.

Such babies seem to become accustomed to the lenses almost at once and show no inclination to try to rub them out of their eyes. The lenses will be put in while the child is anaesthetized. Such lenses have made it possible for the first time in history, for babies with dense congenital cataracts to grow up with something like normal vision.

High refractive errors

People who happen to be extremely short- or long-sighted are much in the same situation as those who have had cataracts removed – in the sense that very strong glasses are needed to bring the eyes into focus. They suffer almost all the optical disadvantages of the post-cataract patient and, of course, enjoy all the same benefits when contact lenses are fitted. High refractive errors are quite common and I think it is a great pity if people in either of these categories are, for any reason, denied the opportunity to experience the remarkable improvement in visual clarity and range that contact lenses can offer them. The advantages are so great that I do not think age should be a consideration and I have fitted both the very young and the very old.

Keratoconus and corneal irregularity

Conical cornea is a fairly rare condition which tends to run in families and in which the person concerned – usually a young man – gradually develops a pointed bulge in the middle of the corneas. In the early stages ordinary spectacles may help, to some extent, but gradually the irregularity in the shape of the corneas gets worse and eventually the vision is quite severely distorted in spite of glasses. Apart from this extraordinary change in the shape of the corneas, the eyes are usually healthy.

If you remember that the reason a contact lens is so efficient is that the lens itself replaces the wrongly curved front surface of the eye by an optically perfect one (see Chapter 2) you will see at once that hard contact lenses are the complete answer to the optical problems of people with keratoconus. The results are excellent and there is some evidence that hard contact lenses actually slow the progress of the disease.

Much commoner than keratoconus is the condition of corneal scarring from injury. Now that the wearing of car seat-belts is mandatory, I expect to see many fewer cases of this, but there are thousands of people whose vision is severely damaged as a result of wounds of the corneas which have healed leaving irregular surfaces. If there are central opaque scars, a contact lens may not help very much, but if the corneas, although irregular, are generally transparent, hard contact lenses can produce an impressive improvement in vision. In such cases contact lenses should always be tried.

Unfortunately, in some cases the shape of the cornea is so abnormal as a result of the injury that it may be difficult, or impossible, to achieve an acceptable contact lens fit. But the attempt should be made.

Astigmatism

We have seen that one of the advantages of hard lenses is that, in most cases of astigmatism they will simply bridge over the difference in the two curves of the cornea so that the effect of the corneal astigmatism is eliminated (see Chapter 2). Astigmatism can, however, occasionally show itself in eyes with properly fitted hard lenses. This is called 'residual astigmatism' and is probably due to the shape of the inside surface of the cornea or of the internal crystalline lens. Normal spherical contact lenses will do nothing to correct such astigmatism, so, if contact lenses are to be worn, the subject must either wear glasses with cylindrical lenses, on top of the contact lenses, or special 'toric' contact lenses. Some major problems are involved both in manufacturing and in fitting these properly. However, a considerable range of toric lenses is now available, both in hard and in soft form.

Bifocal contact lenses for presbyopia

As already mentioned, contact lens wearers who cannot do their own accommodating (near focusing) can simply use reading glasses, on top of their contact lenses. But as the distance error will have been corrected by the contact lenses, the reading glasses will be of a different power from those used with the naked eyes. This is a perfectly satisfactory system and suits most people very well. But there are some who are determined to be rid of glasses for all purposes and for these, the only possibility is a contact lens which has two different powers of correction – one for distance and a stronger one for near.

Early experimental lenses, for this purpose, had a stronger lower segment just like bifocal spectacles, and the designers hoped that the additional weight of the lower segment would keep it in the dependent position. An improvement on this was to fabricate a complete ring of stronger power all round the central optical zone. Some bifocal lenses have a strong lower-segment and rely on 'truncation' (cutting a slice off the lower edge to give a straight edge which rests on the lower lid) to prevent the lens from rotating.

How does the wearer arrange for the near segment to be in front of the pupil? Surprisingly enough, some people find this to be quite easy. Others find it almost impossible. The answer would seem to be that in those cases in which the lens rests on the edge of the lower lid, control by a slight upward movement of the lower lid, on looking down is quite easy. But if the bottom edge of the lens rests behind the lower lid, you have problems!

Bifocal contact lenses are uncommon and, I think, should be regarded as being still in the experimental stage.

Colour vision defects

If a person with defective colour perception (about 10 per cent of males have some degree of colour insensitivity) wears a tinted contact lens on one eye and keeps both eyes open, and if the lens tint is that of the colour not well perceived (usually red), he will be able to identify colours almost normally. (Incidentally, the eye covered by the tinted lens will be different in colour tone from the other eye – so this application is usually only justified if colour identification is really essential.)

Nystagmus

Nystagmus, or 'wobbly-eyes', a condition usually present from birth, almost always affects vision. But when people with nystagmus require glasses, the situation is complicated by the fact that the position of the eyes, in relation to the centres of the spectacle lenses, is constantly changing. Clearly, contact lenses – which move with the eyes and maintain centration – can be valuable to people with nystagmus. Anyone with this condition, who is also short-sighted or significantly long-sighted should certainly try contact lenses.

Cosmetic lenses

Contact lenses can easily be tinted and almost any colour is available at a small extra cost. Interestingly, the effect of a tinted lens is considerably more apparent to the external observer than it is to the wearer – the observer notes a change in apparent eye colour which is about twice as deep as the wearer would expect. The reason for this is that the colouring of the light, seen by the wearer, occurs during only one passage through the tinted lens, whereas the illumination of the iris, as seen by the observer, is by light that has passed through twice. It is important to appreciate this when selecting a tint – the effect will always be greater than you expect. Tinted contact lenses are much used by stage, film and television actors and they are popular too with the general public. It is possible to have a range of tints to suit changing fancy!

A more serious cosmetic application for contact lenses is, however, in the improvement of the appearance of people with disfiguring, white corneal scars, usually from injury or disease but sometimes of congenital origin. Dense corneal scars of this kind (often mistakenly confused with cataract) interfere so seriously with normal eye contact in social intercourse, as to be a source of embarrassment and distress. Tinted contact lenses, sometimes with a simulated pupil, can make a great improvement. Such eyes are usually blind or very poorly sighted so the black-out effect of a deeply tinted lens is no disadvantage.

In some cases the patient, who may, in addition to the social disadvantage, be much troubled by glare from light scatter (especially when driving at night) will find that a lens of this kind offers, also, a notable benefit in comfort and even visual sharpness.

Lenses can be made which are a close match to the normal eye (but, if this is of a light colour, the fixity in the size of the pupil may be noticeable). Alternatively, the patient can wear fairly deeply-tinted contact lenses in both eyes. Incidentally, cosmetic soft lenses, made by sandwiching a thin, coloured sheet between two layers of HEMA (see page 70), are available, and some manufacturers will tint normally soft lenses.

Low visual aid

A limited number of people suffering from severely defective vision find benefit in wearing magnifying telescopic glasses; these are heavy, clumsy and very unsightly. The optical principle of these telescopes is very simple: they consist of a strong negative lens as the eye piece and a strong positive lens as the objective.

There is, however, an alternative which is sometimes preferred and that is to supply the strong negative lens in the form of a contact lens and to use this in conjunction with a normal pair of glasses containing strong plus lenses. The obvious disadvantage is that the eye piece lens can move relative to the objective in the spectacle frame. Nevertheless, some patients, to whom magnification is of real value, have found that they greatly preferred this system and learned to keep the eyes still and to move the head only. Unfortunately, in general, low visual aids have a limited value and perhaps only about 10 per cent of people with severely defective vision find that they offer any worthwhile advantage.

Bandage lenses

Eye specialists often use very thin, high water content soft lenses to treat diseases and injuries to the corneas. These are called 'bandage lenses' and generally have a water content of over 70 per cent and a thickness of about 0.1 mm. Oxygen transfer is almost unimpeded, so the lenses can usually be left in, day and night, for weeks or months.

There are certain very painful corneal conditions in which even the touch of the eyelids causes great distress, and these can be magically relieved by bandage lenses. Corneal ulcers will often heal more rapidly than normal under bandage lenses; incidentally vision is often improved. Various 'dry-eye' conditions, in which tear secretion is inadequate, can be greatly helped and, in lid disorders – with inturning lashes – bandage lenses can provide excellent protection while surgical treatment is being arranged.

These lenses also have application in the emergency management of severe injury, including laceration of the cornea and have sometimes been found helpful after surgical operations such as the sewing up of corneal wounds or even corneal grafting.

10

Technology: Materials and Design

In spite of notable developments in the selection and synthesis of new materials for hard contact lenses, the enormous majority of lenses are still made of the original material PMMA. Polymethyl methacrylate is an acrylic plastic, commonly known as 'Perspex' (this is the trade name for PMMA cast in sheets and first produced in 1933 just in time to be used for aircraft canopies in the Second World War). In many respects it is an ideal material for contact lenses. It has outstanding optical properties, is light weight and can take a high polish. PMMA is a good example of the class of synthetic materials known as 'polymers', meaning 'of many parts'. Each of the 'parts' is a molecule called a monomer and the polymer is made by persuading these molecules to join together in a long chain – 'polymerisation'. The monomers do not, however, simply form chains. They also join together by 'cross-linkage' and the properties of the material largely depends on how frequently these occur. The monomers are not always of one type only, and valuable new materials can be made by polymerising more than one type into the same chain. These materials are called 'co-polymers'.

Originally, PMMA lenses were made by putting a blank of the material into a small automatic turning lathe and carving them out with steel cutters. But now there is a tendency to produce them by polymerising the material inside moulds of high accuracy. One major manufacturer has produced hundreds of quartz glass moulds within which perfect lenses of complex parabolic design, are turned out by this process.

The material from which most soft lenses are made is, surprisingly enough, very similar to PMMA. It too, is a polymer and is called Hydroxyethylmethacrylate, the 'hydro' bit being water.

There is, in fact, only a quite small difference in the monomer, but one which allows molecules of water to link on to the chains. Because the number of cross-linkages between the long chains is small (only about 1 per 200 monomers) there is plenty of room for the water and the material, when fully hydrated, swells up considerably. It is usually called HEMA.

Contact lenses are fabricated from this material in two ways. The first is to start with a button of the completely dry material and to machine and polish it into the shape of a contact lens, being careful to keep even the smallest trace of water well away from the process. When the finished dry lens is put in water it swells up to about twice the original size and becomes very soft and flexible. You can imagine the problems involved in getting the final dimensions right!

The other method is called 'spin-casting'. The monomer and the solvent are mixed together at a temperature below zero (which prevents polymerisation) and are then put into a bowl-shaped mould which is spun rapidly on a spindle. The temperature is then raised to about 65°C and the material, which has been spread out into the proper shape by centrifugal force undergoes polymerisation. By varying the shape of the bowl and the speed of rotation, all sorts of lens shapes can be produced. If the mould is spun very rapidly, the centre of the lens will be thinner than the edge (which is what we need for short sight correction). If the rotation is slower, gravity will ensure that the centre of the lens will be thicker than the edge ('plus' lens for long sight). After polymerisation is complete the lens is put into water to swell to its normal size and shape.

Cellulose Acetate Butyrate

However, PMMA and HEMA are by no means the only materials from which contact lenses can be made. A good deal of fuss was made in the late 1970s about the so-called 'gas permeable' hard lens. The material of which these lenses are made is cellulose actetate butyrate (CAB) a tough plastic used for screw-driver handles (when it is usually stained yellow) but capable of good optical properties.

Probably the main advantage of CAB is that it is much easier to keep wet than PMMA, so the flow of tears under it is improved. It is tough and quite difficult to break. In general, lenses made of CAB are more comfortable than those made of PMMA and the rate of adaptation is usually greater. But nothing in life is perfect, and the surfaces of CAB lenses are noticeably softer and more liable to scratching than PMMA, do not give quite such good vision, absorb some water and sometimes change shape a little, and they are more expensive. Nowadays, the manufacturing tolerances of CAB lenses have improved and fitters can order CAB instead of PMMA for many designs of lenses. Very thin CAB lenses, however, are not satisfactory as they tend to warp. Also, cleaning of CAB lenses must be done even more carefully than with PMMA. Whereas PMMA lenses can be stored dry, CAB lenses must be treated in much the same way as soft lenses and kept constantly in soakage solution when not being worn. Dried CAB lenses suffer a significant change in dimensions. CAB lenses can be useful for patients who, after a long period of satisfactory wear of PMMA lenses, begin to develop intolerance.

Silicone rubber

At first sight, lenses made from this remarkable material seem to have every quality a contact lens should have. They are brilliantly transparent, very flexible (you can stretch them and let them snap back, with perfect safety), they are soft, yet rigid enough to bridge over quite a degree of astigmatism, they are practically indestructible, apparently do not age, and the material is completely non-irritating. Above all, the material is so readily permeable to oxygen that there are no problems in ensuring that the cornea gets its needed supply – even with the eyes closed.

When silicone rubber contact lenses first appeared it seemed that this was the last word and that we would never want anything better. But there was a snag. The very property which makes silicones biologically so inactive turned out to be the big disadvantage for contact lenses. Silicones are water-repellant and non-wettable. The manufacturers have spent millions of pounds trying to make silicone rubber wettable. Their attempts have, so far, produced a surface which initially seems to be satisfactory but after a wearing period of a few months or a year, reverts to the natural characteristic of the material. Silastic lenses which have lost their wettability are very poor optical devices. And they cause a good deal of discomfort.

Co-Polymers

The idea of mixing silicones with other monomers to make a co-polymer combining the properties of both has been taken up by many contact lens producers. One of the most successful is called the 'Boston' material. This is a stable material with about three times the oxygen permeability of CAB but with much less liability to scratching. The wettability is superior to that of PMMA.

Another more recent co-polymer is a material called 'Anduran'. This is a polymer blend of CAB and ethyl-vinylacetate which together produce a hard, but flexible and dimensionally stable material from which lenses can be made which have excellent optical properties and are more wettable than pure CAB.

The contemporary soft lens scene

While the great majority of soft lenses are made of HEMA, this is now usually combined with other monomers such as vinyl-pyrollidone. Other soft lenses contain monoethyl ether methacrylate and dimethyl acrylamide. From that small list of materials is made the majority of lenses sold.

Regrettably, the proportion of soft to hard lenses being worn appears to be rising, especially in Australia (80 per cent) and USA (50 per cent). So far, the British appear to be showing better sense (30 per cent) but this figure is rising too.

Undeniably, however, soft lenses are much easier and quicker to fit than hard and the person who supplies them is likely to have fewer short-term problems with his patients.

Which lenses should I choose?

It would be interesting to try to produce a kind of consumers' guide to contact lenses but, as I have explained, it is the choice of the most suitable lens for each particular patient that matters – rather than any inherent characteristic of the lens. When you pay the bill, you are not paying primarily for the lenses but for the time and expertise of the fitter. Charges may range from three to about six times the wholesale cost of the lenses, the ratio being, quite properly, higher for hard lenses, which require more skill and time.

The wholesale cost of lenses, of any one general type, obviously varies somewhat from one manufacturer to another, but the variations are comparatively small, so the real differences in cost to the customer arise from the variation in the amount charged, by different fitters, for what ought to be the same service. The quality of this service is not easy to evaluate, and prospective customers must simply try to make their own judgement as to the competence and conscientiousness of the fitter. I have given some useful guidance on this in Chapter 4.

Having said that, I would not wish it to be thought that all contact lenses, of any particular type, are equally good, or that the customer should be indifferent to which particular manufacturer's lenses he or she proposes to acquire. I think the customer is entitled to enquire into this and to be rightly suspicious if the fitter tries to brush the matter aside. There is something to be said for choosing a fitter who openly advertises the names of the manufacturers of the lenses he supplies; for there is every reason to suppose that you may safely rely upon the quality and design of lenses from the major manufacturers. No manufacturer can afford to produce an inherently defective product and the broad principles of lens design have long been established. Good fitters will often use lenses from more than one source for, as patients vary so much in their fitting requirements it may not be possible to find the ideal lenses for every patient from the range of one particular maker. In general, fitters who are equipped to do this are probably able to provide a better service than those who use products from one source only.

It would be quite impossible to list, and compare, the whole available range of contact lenses, and I would not wish to try. But I think it might be helpful to mention a few of the major sources, with brief comments, so that the reader may have some basis for judgement. My apologies to those I have failed to mention – this is in no way intended to imply inferiority.

Wohlk Contact Lenses

Wohlk is one of the largest and best-established manufacturers of contact lenses in Europe, supplying millions of lenses annually from a substantial range of lens designs in both hard and soft materials and constantly researching into yet more new designs and materials. The PMMA Parabolar range of lenses have been fitted for many years now and are worn successfully by millions. This range may also be obtained in CAB. In 1981, Wohlk introduced a new gas-permeable, flexible hard lens, of new design, made by a moulding process, from a new co-polymer called Anduran. By the end of 1982, about 40 per cent of Wohlk's production had shifted from PMMA to CAB and Anduran. Anduran lenses are called 'Conflex'. They give excellent wearing time and are quickly tolerated. They may be said to bridge the gap between hard and soft lenses. Other special lenses available from Wohlk include lenses for astigmatism, multifocal lenses, lenses of various colours with either a clear or a tinted pupil for cosmetic purposes, and lenses containing prisms.

Wohlk also have a good range of HEMA soft lenses including some exceptionally thin lenses (Hydroflex SD). The standard 'Hydroflex' lenses have a water content of 40 per cent but Wohlk have, more recently, introduced a lens, called 'Welflex' which is of 65 per cent water content and is intended for patients who have had cataract operations. The Hydroflex range of soft lenses covers several design types and enables a wide range of patients to be fitted.

Coopervision Ltd

Coopervision make 'Permalens', a soft lens of 71 per cent water which allows exceptional oxygen transfer, and which was designed for extended wear. The material from which these lenses is made is called 'Perfilcon A' (a terpolymer of 2-hydroxyethyl methacrylate, N-vinyl-2-pyrolidone and methacrylic acid, with ethylene glycol dimethacrylate as a cross-linking agent, if you really want to know!) Permalenses may, under supervision, be worn continuously, but it is recommended that they are removed monthly for cleaning. Should there be any deterioration in vision or any other obvious symptoms, it is important that the lenses should be removed at once, and advice sought. They should *not* be worn by anyone with any disease of the corneas or conjunctivas, or with tear deficiency or any allergy, or sensitivity to the constituents of soft contact lens solutions.

American Medical Optics

The latest offering from this firm is the 'Sauflon 70' lens, made from 'Lidofilcon A' which has the advantage of combining high water content (70 per cent) and high tensile strength. The strength is said to be superior to that of a normal HEMA lens of 37 per cent water content. Other Sauflon lenses are available from this major manufacturer.

Bausch & Lomb

These are the 'Soflens' people with a large share of the world market. They offer a very extensive range of soft lenses in a variety of designs, mostly made from a material called 'polymacon' which is a trade name for poly (2-hydroxethly methacrylate) – a very common constituent of soft lenses. Bausch & Lomb have brought out some exceptionally thin lenses which are, at the same time, remarkably strong. Obviously, given that the strength is adequate, the thinner the lenses the better. They also make thin toric lenses, for astigmatism, in a material called 'Hefilcon B' available in 1640 different combinations of sphere and cylinder, and have an excellent range of lenses for patients who have had cataract surgery.

Ciba Vision Care

'Cibasoft', Cibathin' and 'Torisoft' lenses are made from 'Tefilcon' which is our old friend HEMA again. All that you have learned about soft lenses apply to these. Ciba also make 'Softint' lenses which are coloured light blue so as to be easier to see in liquid.

Averlan Company Ltd

This is a young and innovative British company which, in the last few years, has made substantial developments in design and manufacturing technology, especially in hard lenses. It now offers a good range of lenses which can be supplied, on order, in a variety of materials including PMMA, CAB, P.S.1 ('Boston') and 'Boston Two'. These 'Boston' materials are co-polymers of silicon and PMMA, and offer about three times the oxygen transmission of CAB. One of the most interesting features of the Averlan output is the range of 'Ultra-thin Flexible Lenses'. These are very small and exceedingly thin, hard lenses with which good centring and comfort can be obtained in patients otherwise difficult to fit. They are of such small diameter that a considerable proportion of the corneal surface is left exposed to the atmosphere, thereby improving direct oxygen access.

Averlan's latest product is 'Hypergas 2000' which is said to be a 'revolution in patient comfort and lens technology'. These new lenses are said to be much less fragile than ordinary gas-permeable lenses, to be hard-wearing and dimensionally stable, and to be flexible, comfortable and of high oxygen permeability. They can, in many cases be made very thin, so as to improve further the transmission of oxygen and CO_2.

Other suppliers

Considerations of space preclude more than a bare mention of some of the other major suppliers, such as the very large European manufacturer Titmus-Eurocon who, along with Wohlk, did much of the early developmental work on HEMA polymers and lens designs; Contact Lens Manufacturing, Ltd., of London; Hydron Europe, Ltd.; Hydron Australia, Ltd.; Smith and Nephew, Ltd.; Soft Lenses, Inc., of California; Aquaflex Contact Lens Products, of New York; Wesley Jesston of Chicago and The Toyo Contact Lens Company of Nagoya, Japan. All these are major international manufacturers of Hydrogel Contact Lenses. Many other firms, small and large, have broken into this lucrative market in recent years, and the resultant intense competition is very much in the interests of the public. For, with such a proliferation of materials and designs, there are now few patients who may not be satisfactorily fitted, given that the practitioner is ready to spend the necessary time and take the necessary trouble.

11

Quick Answers to Common Questions

Most of these questions are dealt with, at greater length, in the appropriate chapters of this book, but this quick reference section might be useful.

Q. Are contact lenses better than glasses?
A. For people who need to wear glasses all the time, definitely yes.

Q. Why?
A. Better and more natural vision, wider visual field, comfortable ears, no coffee fog, no problems in rain, cosmetically advantageous.

Q. Do they hurt?
A. No. Not unless something is very wrong.

Q. Can anyone wear contact lenses?
A. A small proportion of people are temperamentally unsuitable.

Q. I mean, do some people have unsuitable eyes?
A. Only if the eyes are diseased. Even then, some can benefit from contact lenses, if they are prescribed by a specialist.

Q. Are contact lenses suitable for sport?
A. Yes, for most sports, very. But you will probably lose them if you swim in them.

QUICK ANSWERS TO COMMON QUESTIONS

Q. What about tennis?

A. Yes. But soft lenses may be better than hard ones.

Q. Do you advise hard or soft lenses?

A. Hard lenses should always be tried first. You should try soft lenses only if you cannot be satisfactorily fitted with hard ones.

Q. Why?

A. Because hard lenses are safer, much longer-lasting, optically better, cheaper and easier to keep clean.

Q. Can I wear hard lenses occasionally only?

A. No.

Q. Why not?

A. You must gradually build up tolerance and this means wearing them every day.

Q. Can I wear soft lenses on an occasional basis?

A. Yes. But if you need to wear them, why not wear them constantly?

Q. Can I leave hard lenses in all the time?

A. No.

Q. What about soft lenses?

A. Normal soft lenses, no. Special very thin and/or those of high water content can be worn continuously, under close supervision.

Q. Do you recommend these for people with ordinary short sight?

A. No.

Q. Why not?

A. They are very expensive, usually short-lived, often become spoiled and can cause corneal damage.

Q. Are soft lenses much more comfortable than hard ones?
A. A person who has adapted to hard lenses would notice very little difference. The immediate comfort is greater with soft lenses.

Q. Why?
A. Mainly because they are larger and have a more effectively wetted front surface.

Q. So it isn't because the material is softer?
A. No. The main discomfort comes from the upper eyelid margin striking the upper edge of the hard lens. This is impossible with large soft lenses. Small soft lenses are quite uncomfortable.

Q. Are hard lenses made of glass?
A. Never! Glass is too heavy, too fragile and too dangerous.

Q. What are hard lenses made of?
A. Perspex. Commonly known as polymethylmethacrylate. Some are made of a more wettable material called CAB, or of more recently developed materials.

Q. Is CAB better than PMMA?
A. Yes and no. It wets better and you may build up wearing time quicker. But CAB is softer and is more easily scratched.

Q. Should hard lenses be stored dry or wet?
A. Wet.

Q. What would happen if I put dry lenses on my eyes?
A. I expect you would want to take them off again very quickly!

QUICK ANSWERS TO COMMON QUESTIONS

Q. Would they do any harm?
A. Probably not, but they would be very uncomfortable.

Q. Should I suck them?
A. No.

Q. Why not?
A. Your mouth contains, and can tolerate, quite a range of germs that could infect your eyes.

Q. I tried hard lenses and failed. Will soft lenses be suitable for me?
A. Probably. But perhaps the fit of the hard lens wasn't quite right. There are several possible reasons for failure apart from yourself!

Q. Why should I have to pay so much for a couple of little bits of plastic?
A. Contact lenses are miracles of optical perfection, but most of what you pay is a fee for the fitter's skill, knowledge, time and overheads.

Q. Can I insure contact lenses?
A. Certainly. There are many different schemes of insurance. Premiums are not high.

Q. How long will it take me to reach all-day wear with hard lenses?
A. This varies quite a lot. Usually three to four weeks, but some people never achieve all-day wear.

Q. What about soft lenses?
A. Usually adjustment is much quicker – as little as a week in many cases.

Q. Will my eyes be continuously red?
A. If they are, something is wrong. Contact the fitter at once.

Q. Can you tell that someone is wearing contact lenses?
A. Usually not.

Q. Can they be coloured?
A. Yes. Lenses can be tinted almost any colour.

Q. Is that expensive?
A. No.

Q. I'm worried about lenses slipping round behind my eyes. Does this often happen?
A. No, never, It's impossible!

Q. I need glasses for reading only. Would I be suitable for contact lenses?
A. No. Stick to your glasses.

Q. I have astigmatism. Does this mean I can't wear contact lenses?
A. Not at all. Hard lenses cover astigmatism. It is even possible to have special soft lenses for astigmatism.

Q. What is spectacle blur?
A. Temporarily blurred vision in glasses after wearing contact lenses.

Q. Is that serious?
A. No. Not unless very severe and persistent.

Q. What causes it?
A. Either a moulding of your corneas into a new shape, or a slight swelling from accumulation of fluid in the corneal outer layer.

Q. My friend wears very thin, hard lenses. Is that a good idea?
A. The smaller the better, so long as they give good vision.

Q. She says she never gets spectacle blur. Why is that?
A. Very small lenses are less liable to cause this, because the corneas have a better oxygen supply.

Q. Why is oxygen important?
A. Corneas, like all living tissues, need oxygen to survive. As they can't get it via the blood because they do not contain blood vessels, they have to get it direct from the atmosphere.

Q. What happens if I get a bit of grit behind a contact lens?
A. You will know all about it. This doesn't happen often.

Q. What should I do?
A. Take out the lens and wash it.

Q. But suppose the grit stays in my eye?
A. Get someone to remove it with the corner of a clean handkerchief, or see your doctor. Don't use your lenses meantime.

Q. Is it very difficult to insert and remove contact lenses?
A. The difficulties in insertion are largely psychological. Removing lenses is easy, but it takes a bit of practice to learn to do it quickly.

Q. Is it a good idea to use a rubber sucker to remove lenses?
A. No. Not unless you can be certain that the lens is on the cornea.

Q. Are suckers useful for inserting lenses?
A. Generally, no. The finger-tip is much better, because it is soft and therefore less likely to cause accidental damage.

Q. Will the fitter teach me to put in and take out the lenses?

A. Certainly. This is part of the service.

Q. I have had cataract operations. Do you think contact lenses are a good idea?

A. Yes. This is one of the strongest indications for contact lenses. You will be amazed at the improvement in vision.

Q. But I'm very nervous about handling the lenses. Could I damage my eyes?

A. Almost impossible. But you will need professional instruction.

Q. I wear soft lenses. What is the best way to keep them clean?

A. Most people use cleaning and soaking solutions and have no trouble. But these contain chemicals that can eventually cause persistent irritation to the eyes or sometimes allergy.

Q. What about make-up?

A. Put in the lenses first.

Q. What about boiling them?

A. Most soft lenses can be safely boiled, but not all, so do check with your fitter before you use this method.

Q. Is boiling a good way to clean lenses?

A. Boiling is completely effective. But you must first be sure that there is no protein or other foreign material on the lenses, as boiling will make this difficult or impossible to remove.

Q. How can I get rid of protein contaminants then?

A. The best way is to use an enzyme cleaner. This comes in tablet form, to be dissolved in water. Follow the instructions.

Q. Why are there so many different kinds of contact lens solutions?

A. There are, essentially, only three kinds – cleaning, wetting and soaking.

Q. Do I need all three kinds?

A. No. You need a cleaner and a soaker. There are various combination solutions and, of course, different solutions for hard and soft lenses.

Q. Can't I use hard lens solutions for soft lenses?

A. No.

Q. Why not?

A. The chemicals in hard lens solutions are in higher concentration and will be absorbed into the soft lenses. These will then be very likely to irritate your eyes.

Q. How should I clean hard lenses?

A. Use cleaning solution after every wear, rinse it off and then soak them overnight in soaking solution. If very dirty, use vinegar or washing-up liquid, then repeat above.

Q. Can I boil hard lenses?

A. No. If you do, you will certainly destroy them!

Q. Can polishing change the power of my lenses?

A. Yes, if excessive.

Q. Could polishing damage my eyes?

A. No, but it might cause a slight sense of 'eye-strain'.

Q. Will my fitter polish my lenses for me?

A. Possibly. Why not ask?

Q. *Can the power of my hard lenses be changed, if I become more short-sighted?*

A. Yes quite easily, if the equipment is to hand. But lens adjustments, and even polishing, are becoming increasingly uneconomic and most fitters will simply order new lenses for you.

Q. *Can the power of soft lenses be changed?*

A. No.

Q. *Why do soft lenses have a limited life?*

A. Surfaces become permanently contaminated or pitted, edges become nicked, lenses tear, material becomes discoloured.

Q. *What will happen if I let my soft lenses dry?*

A. They will turn into little grey potato crisps.

Q. *Does that mean they are ruined?*

A. By no means – unless you snap them. Just put them back into water, or a soaking solution and they will soon be restored to normal.

Q. *What are comfort drops?*

A. These are viscous solutions which help to keep the lenses wetted. They are sometimes helpful in building up wearing time.

Q. *I wear soft lenses. Can I use medical eye drops?*

A. Be careful! The preservative might concentrate in your lens and cause irritation. The active ingredient might also do the same, in which case you will get more than was intended.

Q. *I get hay fever. Is it all right to wear my lenses during an attack?*

A. Between attacks – no problem. During an attack there is a risk of losing lenses if your eyes water or you sneeze much. A specialist could prescribe useful eye-drops.

QUICK ANSWERS TO COMMON QUESTIONS

Q. Can I wear my lenses if I have conjunctivitis?

A. Positively not. And make sure that they, and your lens containers, are sterilized before you wear them again.

Q. How?

A. Thorough cleaning, enzyme and boiling (if safe) for soft lenses; thorough cleaning and prolonged soakage in solution for hard lenses. Don't forget the container!

Q. I have glaucoma. Should I wear contact lenses?

A. Ask your specialist. Sometimes soft lenses are undesirable, but they can be used to improve the delivery of medication.

Q. At what age can contact lenses be fitted?

A. Contact lenses have been successfully fitted to new-born babies, to ninety-year-old post-cataract patients and to people of every age in between.

Q. Yes, but apart from medical indications when should young people start?

A. People with moderate degrees of short sight might start around sixteen years, but if the myopia is severe, an earlier start is justified. But in this case an adult should supervise wearing time and routine cleaning of the lenses.

Q. Do young people have many problems with contact lenses?

A. Young people are remarkably tolerant and have few problems. Those that arise are nearly always due to overwear and lack of cleanliness.

Q. Which kinds of people are least likely to be successful with contact lenses?

A. Males over 40. Teenage girls almost always succeed!

Q. I am short-sighted, 45, and usually take off my glasses to read. Do you recommend contact lenses?

A. No.

Q. *Why not?*

A. You will certainly need to wear reading glasses on top of your lenses.

Q. *I am short-sighted, 50, and need two pairs of glasses. I can't bear the thought of bifocal glasses. Is there any alternative?*

A. Certainly. Contact lenses and reading glasses.

Q. *I am long-sighted, 45, and beginning to have problems reading. Also, my distance vision is sometimes a little blurred. Do you recommend contact lenses?*

A. Yes. They should solve all your problems for a number of years. Eventually, of course, you will need reading glasses as well as contact lenses, but you will be spared bifocals.

Q. *Is it true that contact lenses can prevent short sight from progressing?*

A. No.

Q. *Is it true that short sight can be cured by an operation on the cornea?*

A. The procedures are dangerous and the effect often temporary. Permanent damage may occur. Not recommended.

Q. *Shall I require to change my contact lenses as often as I change my glasses?*

A. No. Much less often. You may save money in the long run.

Q. *I sometimes see double with one eye when wearing my lenses. Is this serious?*

A. This suggests that one lens is not centring properly. Not serious, but you should tell your fitter.

Q. *My vision often fogs up but clears when I blink. What should I do?*

A. Blink more. Contact lens wearers sometimes get into a bad habit of inadequate blinking. Make sure *you* don't!

QUICK ANSWERS TO COMMON QUESTIONS

Q. *Why is it important to put the plug in the sink when washing my lenses?*

A. If you drop the lens you'll never retrieve it!

Q. *Do you recommend tinted lenses?*

A. Yes, but not too deeply tinted. Tinted lenses relieve the light sensitivity that most wearers have, initially. They are also easier to find if dropped in water.

Q. *Can I use a clean tissue to clean my lenses?*

A. No. Tissues always cause scratching.

Q. *What should I use then?*

A. Your finger tips – thoroughly washed first, of course.

Q. *Is it easy to insert contact lenses in someone else's eyes?*

A. Very. Easier than putting them in your own – providing they will keep their eyes open properly.

Q. *My mother has had cataracts removed. Could I learn to put in and remove her contact lenses for her?*

A. Very easily. The specialist will be delighted to instruct you and your mother will bless you!

Q. *What is the difference between an ophthalmic optician and an optometrist?*

A. No difference.

Q. *Who may fit and prescribe contact lenses?*

A. An ophthalmic optician, an ophthalmic medical practitioner or an ophthalmologist.

Q. *What is an ophthalmologist?*

A. A doctor who is a specialist in the disorders of the eye.

Q. *Whom should I see if I have major complications from contact lens wear?*

A. An ophthalmologist. Your family doctor will refer you.

Glossary

ACCOMMODATION
The (unconscious) process of changing the focus of the eyes so that near objects are clearly seen. The internal lens changes its shape automatically. The lenses become rigid with age and accommodation becomes progressively less effective (See PRESBYOPIA).

APHAKIA
An eye without a crystalline lens. This is the state after cataract surgery, if an intraocular implant has not been performed.

ASTIGMATISM
Unevenness in the curvature of the cornea. The top-to-bottom bulge may be more or less steep than the side-to-side one.

BANDAGE LENS
A very thin, high water content, permanent-wear, contact lens, not intended for optical correction, but used as a protective membrane in various diseases and injuries of the cornea.

BENZALKONIUM CHLORIDE
An ammonium compound used as a preservative in contact lens solutions, eye drops etc. It is an effective germicide for hard lenses. Should never be used with soft lenses.

CAB
Cellulose acetate butyrate. A good material for making hard lenses. Wets better than PMMA (Perspex) but is more easily scratched. Said to be permeable to oxygen.

CATARACT
Clouding of the internal lens of the eye. The only remedy is

removal of the lens, which may be replaced by a plastic implant. If not, contact lenses are best, after the operation.

CONJUNCTIVA

A transparent membrane attached around the edge of the cornea and lying loosely on the white of the eye. In the recesses of the lids, the conjunctiva folds forward to form the inner lining of the eyelids, making it impossible for a contact lens to slip back behind the eyeball. Inflammation of the conjunctiva (from any cause) is called conjunctivitis.

CORNEA

The front (external) lens of the eyeball.

CORNEAL ABRASION

A term loosely used to describe localized destruction and loss of corneal epithelium. Commonly caused by overwear of hard lenses. There is acute pain, foreign body sensation and watering and it is very difficult to keep the eye open. Antibiotic drops should be prescribed and the eye otherwise kept shut for 24 to 28 hours.

CORNEAL ULCER

An infected corneal abrasion. This is serious and should be treated by an eye specialist. Tissue destruction extends deeper than the epithelium and a permanent scar results. If the ulcer is central there will be permanent disturbance of vision.

CRYSTALLINE LENS

The internal, fine-focusing, adjustable lens of the eye, changes in the curvature of which enable us to see clearly both distant and near objects. When this lens becomes opaque, the condition is called 'cataract'.

DIOPTRE

A unit of lens power. A 1 dioptre lens has a focal length of

1 metre. A very mildly short-sighted person might need lenses of 1 dioptre. The average need is about 3 dioptres. 'High' myopes might need 10 to 20 dioptres. You can judge the power required, roughly, by dividing 100 cms by the farthest distance in centimetres at which you can see clearly. Thus, if you can see objects clearly at 50 cms, you need 2 dioptre lenses.

DIPLOPIA
Double vision.

ENZYME
A biochemical substance which acts as a catalyst to promote a chemical reaction. Enzyme contact lens cleaners are 'proteolytic', that is, they break down the molecules of protein contamination of soft lenses but without affecting the lenses.

EPITHELIUM
The outer 'skin' of the cornea. This can be damaged fairly easily by lack of oxygen or physical injury, but has a remarkable capacity for speedy regeneration and recovery.

EYE-BALL
(See Chapter 1.) In summary, it is a miniature closed-circuit television camera with a maximum aperture of about f2.8 and a focal length of about 25 mm. Both the light control and the focusing are automatic. The photocells are connected to an internal micro-processor and the output is a multi-channel, frequency-modulated signal. It comes in various sizes and the main lens power does not always correspond exactly to the axial length – hence the need for contact lenses.

FITTING LENSES
These are standard sets of contact lenses used by the fitter to find the most suitable lens for the patient. Both hard and soft fitting lenses are used.

FLUORESCEIN
A harmless dye which fluoresces in ultra-violet light and which can be used to stain the tear film on the cornea and so check the fit of a hard contact lens. It must never be used with soft lenses as it will dye them permanently yellow.

FOCIMETER
An optical instrument for measuring the power of spectacle lenses.

HAPTIC LENSES
A lens, much larger than a normal contact lens, made of plastic or glass, fitting behind the eyelids and with the central optical portion lying over but not necessarily touching the cornea. Very seldom used nowadays.

HEMA
Hydroxyethylmethacrylate. A plastic gel containing from 20 per cent to 80 per cent water. Many soft lenses are made from this material.

HYDROPHILIC
Water-loving. Such substances attract water.

HYDROPHOBIC
Water-repellant.

HYPERMETROPIA
Long sight. Usually causes no problems in young people. Older people can't see near objects clearly and later may need glasses for distance vision also.

KERATOCONUS
Conical cornea. A hereditary disease. The eyes are usually normal until adolescence, then the corneas begin to bulge centrally.

KERATOMETER
An optical instrument used by the contact lens fitter to measure the curves of the cornea.

KERATOPATHY
Any disease of the cornea.

LACRIMAL GLANDS
Tiny buds of tissue which manufacture tears. The main lacrimal glands consist of large collections of these buds and lie under the bone at the upper and outer corner of the eye sockets. These work during weeping or when the eye is irritated. The normal wetness of the eye is provided by *accessory* lacrimal glands lying in the conjunctiva.

LENS
A piece of glass or plastic so shaped as to cause bending of light rays. Lentil shaped. Most commonly found in spectacles but widely used in all sorts of optical devices and, of course, in the form of contact lenses.

MERIDIAN
A line lying on the surface of a curve. Most corneas are a little steeper in the vertical meridian than in the horizontal curve. The meridia of maximal and minimal power are at right angles to each other.

MICRO-ORGANISMS
Living cells (often germs) which, under suitable conditions, can reproduce themselves freely and cause damage to human tissues. Many produce very powerful poisons.

MYOPIA
Short sight. Near objects can be seen clearly. Distant objects look blurred.

GLOSSARY

OEDEMA
A swelling and change of shape caused by accumulation of water in the tissues. Can occur in the cornea as a result of oxygen lack and may seriously affect vision.

OPTICAL DENSITY
Transparent substances (like glass, PMMA, water, cornea etc) slow the velocity of light to different extents and curved interfaces between materials of differing optical density will cause bending of the light rays. The greater the difference in the optical densities, the more acute will be the bending.

OPTIC ZONE
The central, circular part of a contact lens which actually contains the patient's prescription. If this central part is too small, or the lens does not centre properly, the patient may be seeing partly through the optic zone and partly through the periphery, with unsatisfactory visual results.

OVERWEAR SYNDROME
A set of symptoms varying from slight discomfort and mistiness of vision (OEDEMA) to the acute experience of CORNEAL ABRASION (see page 91).

OXYGEN
The most important gas in air. Vital to life. Vital for normal health and clarity of the corneas. The corneas obtain oxygen direct from the atmosphere via the tear film.

PHOTOCELL
In engineering, this is a device which, when light falls upon it, gives out a small electrical current. The photocells in the retina are called rods and cones and are extremely sensitive to light. The cones are sensitive to colour.

PMMA
Polymethylmethacrylate. Perspex. Most hard contact lenses are made from perspex – never from glass.

PRESBYOPIA
Distance vision remains normal, but the person concerned can no longer bring near objects into focus. Usually comes on around age of 45. Gets gradually worse until about 60.

PRESCRIPTION
The optical power of a spectacle, or contact lens required to compensate for long sight, short sight, astigmatism and presbyopia.

RADIUS
The distance from the centre of a circle to the edge. The steepness of the curves of corneas are expressed as radii, in millimetres. Very steep corneas may have a radius of less than 7 mm. Flat corneas have radii of up to 8.5 mm. A radius between these two figures is commonly found.

RADIUS OF CURVATURE
Optical surfaces (such as the outside of the cornea or the front or back of a contact lens) must often be measured. The degree of curvature is expressed as the distance from the centre to the surface of the sphere with the same degree of curvature. This is the radius of the sphere. A short radius sphere has a very steeply curved surface and a long radius sphere is larger, with a correspondingly flatter surface.

REFRACTION
Literally, bending of light rays. The word is commonly used for the eye test by which the optician discovers the lenses needed to correct the patient's short sight, long sight or astigmatism.

GLOSSARY

SILASTIC

Silicone rubber. A remarkable material from which brilliantly transparent lenses can be made. These lenses allow free transmission of oxygen to the cornea. The major disadvantage is the difficulty of achieving and maintaining the wettability of the surface. Very strong. Would be the ideal material for contact lenses if the surface could be made permanently wettable.

SQUINT

The condition in which only one eye looks directly at the object of interest. The other eye looks elsewhere and the vision must be 'turned off' or double vision is experienced.

TEAR FILM

Essential for corneal health and clear vision. Has three layers (mucin, salt water and oil) and all must be normal for satisfactory comfort and vision.

TEST TYPE

A vision testing chart which must be used at a fixed distance from the patient (normally 6 metres, sometimes 5 metres) and which must have standard letters and be suitably illuminated. Special test type is also used for near vision.

THIOMERSAL

A mercurial compound used as an antiseptic in contact lens soakage solutions. Sometimes called *Thimerosal*, it may become a cause of chronic irritation in long-term soft contact lens wearers.

TORIC

A surface having curves of two different radii, like the side of an egg or a rugby ball. Toric lenses produce, or correct, astigmatism.

TRIAL FRAME

A pair of adjustable spectacles with slots into which various lenses can be fitted for testing purposes.

Index

Overcoming Common Problems
MAIL ORDER FORM

THE ABC OF EATING   *Joy Melville*
Coping with anorexia, bulimia and   cased **£6.95** ☐
compulsive eating   paper **£2.50** ☐

AN A–Z OF ALTERNATIVE MEDICINE
Brent Hafen and Kathryn Frandsen   cased **£6.95** ☐
     paper **£2.50** ☐

ARTHRITIS   *Dr William Fox*
Is your suffering really necessary?   paper **£2.50** ☐

BIRTH OVER THIRTY   *Sheila Kitzinger*   cased **£6.95** ☐
     paper **£2.50** ☐

BODY LANGUAGE   *Allan Pease*   cased **£7.95** ☐
     paper **£2.95** ☐

CALM DOWN   *Dr Paul Hauck*
How to cope with frustration and anger   paper **£2.50** ☐

DEPRESSION   *Dr Paul Hauck*   cased **£6.95** ☐
     paper **£2.50** ☐

DIVORCE AND SEPARATION
Angela Willans   cased **£6.95** ☐
Everywoman's guide to a new life   paper **£2.50** ☐

ENJOYING MOTHERHOOD
Dr Brice Pitt
How to have a happy pregnancy   paper **£2.50** ☐

THE EPILEPSY HANDBOOK
Shelagh McGovern   paper **£3.95** ☐

FAMILY FIRST AID   *Dr Andrew Stanway* paper **£3.95** ☐

SOLVING YOUR PERSONAL PROBLEMS
Peter Honey   cased **£6.95** ☐
                                           paper **£2.50** ☐

STRESS AND YOUR STOMACH
Dr Vernon Coleman   paper **£2.50** ☐

SUCCESSFUL SEX   *Dr F.E. Kenyon*   paper **£2.50** ☐

WHAT EVERYONE SHOULD KNOW   cased **£6.50** ☐
ABOUT DRUGS   *Kenneth Leech*   paper **£2.50** ☐

WHY BE AFRAID?   *Dr Paul Hauck*   paper **£2.50** ☐

All these books can be ordered direct by post. Just tick the titles you want and fill in the form below.

Name ....

Address ....

....

....

Write to OCP Mail Order, SPCK, Marylebone Road, London NW1 4DU.

Please enclose remittance to the value of the cover price plus:

UK: 50p for the first book plus 32p per copy for each additional book ordered.

Overseas: 75p for the first book plus 45p per copy for each additional book.

Sheldon Press reserve the right to show new retail prices on covers which may differ from those previously advertised in the text or elsewhere. Postage rates are also subject to revision.